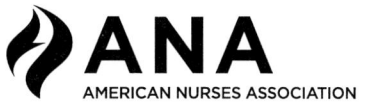

Safe Patient Handling and Mobility

Interprofessional National Standards
Across the Care Continuum

American Nurses Association
Silver Spring, Maryland
2021

The American Nurses Association (ANA) is a national professional association. This ANA publication—*Safe Patient Handling and Mobility: Interprofessional National Standards Across the Care Continuum*—reflects the thinking of the practice specialty of holistic nursing on various issues and should be reviewed in conjunction with state board of nursing policies and practices. State law, rules, and regulations govern the practice of nursing, while *Safe Patient Handling and Mobility: Interprofessional National Standards Across the Care Continuum* guides nurses in the application of their professional skills and responsibilities.

American Nurses Association
8515 Georgia Avenue, Suite 400
Silver Spring, MD 20910-3492
1-800-274-4ANA
www.NursingWorld.org

ISBN: Print: 978-1-953985-20-0   SAN: 851-3481
ePDF: 978-1-953985-21-7
ePUB: 978-1-953985-22-4
Mobi: 978-1-953985-23-1

First printing: October 2021

Contents

Contributors

The American Nurses Association wishes to thank everyone who generously contributed their valuable time and expertise to the development of the 2nd Edition of the *Safe Patient Handling and Mobility: Interprofessional National Standards Across the Care Continuum*. This resource builds on and replaces the previous edition of the *Safe Patient Handling and Mobility: Interprofessional National Standards Across the Care Continuum*. We could not have accomplished such a comprehensive document without you!

STANDARDS ADVISORY GROUP

Lynda Enos, RN, MS, COHN-S, CPE,
HumanFit, LLC

Susan Gallagher, PhD, MSN, MA, RN, CBN,
Celebration Institute

Mary Matz, MSPH, CPE, CSPHP,
Patient Care Ergonomics Solutions, LLC

Vicki J. Missar, MS, CPE, SSBB, CSPHP, CHSP,
Aon Risk Solutions

Renee Neidhardt, MSN, RN,
Charlie Norwood VA Medical Center

Patti Wawzyniecki, MS, CSPHP

STANDARDS WORK GROUP

Colin J. Brigham, CIH, CSP, CPE, CPEA, CSPHP, FAIHA,
TRC Companies, Inc.

Shannon Gallagher,
Patient Positioning Systems, LLC (PPS)

Dee Kumpar, MBA, BSN, RN,
HD Nursing

Manon Labreche, PT, CEAS II,
Tampa General Hospital

Kelsey McCoskey, MS, OTR/L, CPE, CSPHP,
US Army Public Health Center

Andrea McKinney, MHA, MA, OT, CIE,
Eye on Ergonomics Inc.

Todd R. Mohrmann, MA,
Dynamic Training, Inc.

Renee Neidhardt, MSN, RN,
Charlie Norwood VA Medical Center

Carrie L. Norcutt, MSN, RN-BC, PHN, CBN,
Ensign Group, Inc. Villa Maria Post-Acute (Santa Maria, CA)

Mary J. Ogg, MSN, RN, CNOR

Leslie Pickett, PT, DPT, CPE,
BETA Healthcare Group

Lisa Pompeii, PhD, MS, RN, FAAOHN

Asha Roy, OTD, OTR/L, MBA, MS, MAS PSHQ, CSPHP,
Northwell Health, New York

Susan Salsbury, BS, OTR/L, CDMS, CSPHP,
OhioHealth System

Christina Squires, MSN, RN, CSPHP,
Dignity Health Central Coast Service Area, CA

Rhonda Turner, RN, MSN-LD, CSPHA,
Banner Health, Northern Colorado Medical Center

Kimberly D. Waltrip, PhD, APRN-BC,
Western Governors University

Eric A. Williams, MD, MS, MMM, FAAP, FCCM,
Texas Children's Hospital

ANA STAFF

Ruth Francis, MPH, MCHES—ANA Staff Lead
Carol Bickford, PhD, RN-BC, CPHIMS, FAMIA, FHIMSS, FAAN
Katie Boston-Leary, PhD, MHA, MBA, RN, NEA-BC
Kendra McMillian, RN, MPH
Erin Walpole, PMP
James Angelo, MA

ABOUT THE AMERICAN NURSES ASSOCIATION

The American Nurses Association (ANA) is the premier organization representing the interests of the nation's 4.2 million registered nurses. ANA advances the profession by fostering high standards of nursing practice, promoting a safe and ethical work environment, bolstering the health and wellness of nurses, and advocating on health care issues that affect nurses and the public. ANA is at the forefront of improving the quality of health care for all. For more information visit www.nursingworld.org.

ACKNOWLEDGEMENT

We would like to recognize the importance and extent of the Veterans Health Administration's (VHA) support in facilitating SPHM in the United States (US). The VHA SPHM Program and resources were the drivers for SPHM acceptance throughout the US. Without VHA support, ANA would not have made as much progress in the SPHM arena as it has. Specifically, we want to thank the three VHA staff who were responsible for the initiation and success of the original VHA SPHM Program.

Michael Hodgson, MD, MPH, for his momentous support of SPHM in the VHA where he was the Chief Consultant, Occupational Health and the Director, Occupational Health Program, Veterans Health Administration from 1999 – 2012. Dr. Hodgson's dedication, leadership, intellectual support, and tenacity in obtaining financial support for SPHM research, VA program leadership, and the national VA SPHM program made possible the development and unrestricted dissemination to other organizations of VA SPHM resources, research findings, and knowledge gained through the system wide SPHM program implementation in over 150 VA facilities.

Audrey Nelson, PhD, RN, FAAN, Director, Patient Safety Center of Inquiry, for taking on the difficult task of determining how patient handling injuries could be reduced through technology and programmatic efforts; conducting influential SPHM research studies; initiating annual SPHM conferences; facilitating development of general, bariatric, orthopedic, and perioperative SPHM tools for SPHM, and forging many other SPHM initiatives that are too numerous to note.

Mary Matz, MSPH, CPE, CSPHP, for her tenacity in leading, driving, and managing the original VHA SPHM program; ensuring over 150 VHA facilities were equipped to conduct safe patient handling and mobility; ensuring over 150 VHA Facility Coordinators and thousands of Peer Leaders were educated in SPHM, technology, and program facilitators; disseminating VHA lessons learned to the ANA, OSHA, NIOSH, and other national organizations and educational institutions; and educating design professionals in SPHM, ultimately generating national criteria for the design and construction of healthcare facilities.

Throughout the Standards, readers will find resources and references from the VHA, from Dr. Audrey Nelson, Mary Matz, and other VHA personnel. The original, and this second edition of the SPHM Standards, are direct outcomes of the dedication and efforts of these three noted above and other VHA SPHM leaders. We thank you!

The Continuing Need for Safe Patient Handling and Mobility (SPHM) Standards

Are healthcare workers still being needlessly injured at work?

Workers in many healthcare occupations continue to suffer a higher rate of musculoskeletal disorders (MSDs) involving days away from work than workers in many other industries (Bureau of Labor Statistics [BLS], November 2020 and 2019; Figure 1).

In 2018, The Bureau of Labor Statistics (BLS) data showed that 'Health care and social assistance' lost-time injuries involving MSDs were second only to 'Transportation and warehousing' with other seemingly more hazardous industries having fewer lost-time injuries (BLS, May 2020; Figure 2).

In 2019, Emergency medical technicians and paramedics, and Nursing assistants, orderlies, and psychiatric aides continued to have the highest rates of strain

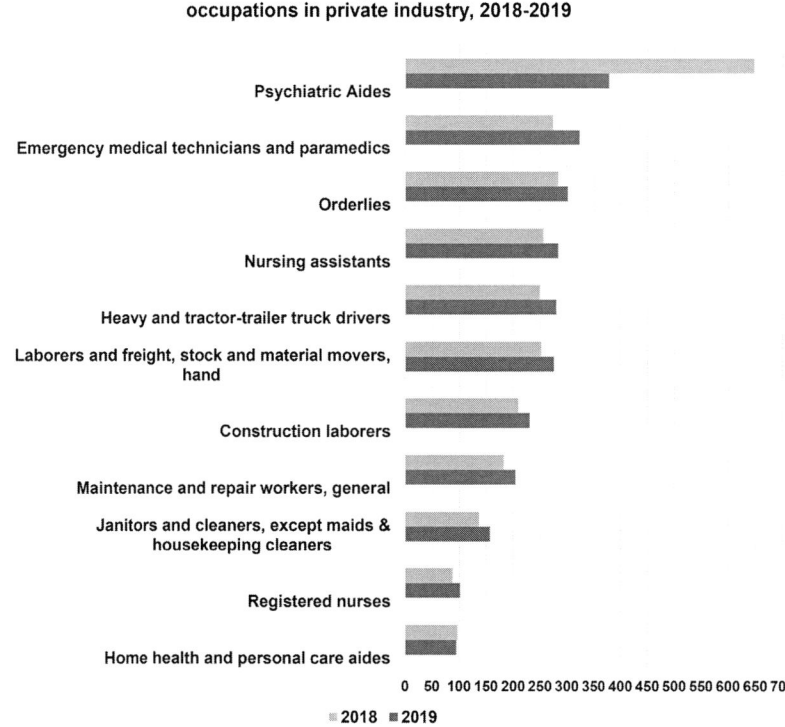

Figure 1. 2018 and 2019 Incidence rates of cases involving days away from work for selected occupations in the private industry, per 10,000 full-time workers (BLS November 2020 and BLS 2019).

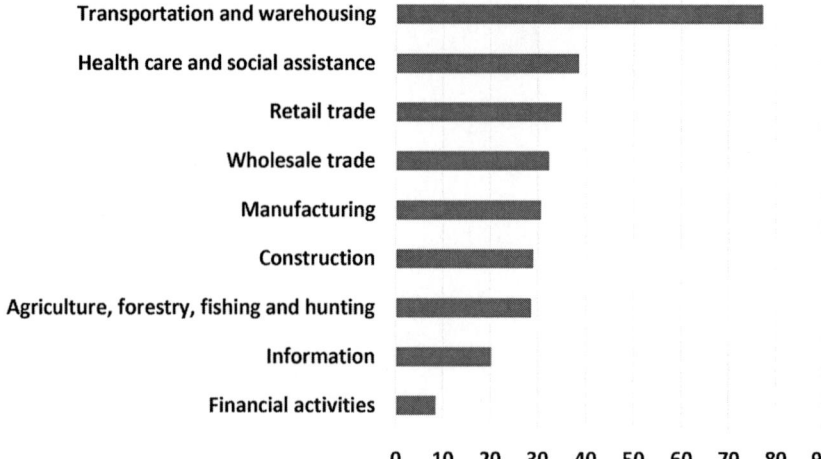

Incidence rate of days away from work of injuries and illnesses involving musculoskeletal disorders by selected industries, US, private sector, 2018

Figure 2. 2018 Incidence rates of days away from work for injuries and illnesses involving musculoskeletal disorders by selected industries, United States, private sector, per 10,000 full-time workers (BLS, May 2020).

and sprain injuries associated with lifting and lowering activities of all healthcare-related occupations (BLS, November 2020).

The costs associated with these injuries were and are significant. In 2018, costs of overexertion-related injuries from outside sources (handling objects – including healthcare consumers) were 2.06 billion dollars and accounted for 38.5% of the direct costs of all worker compensation claims with more than 5 days away from work in healthcare and social assistance industries (Liberty Mutual Insurance, 2021).

According to the 2018–2019 Healthy Nurse Healthy Nation® (HNHN) survey, 58% of nurse respondents indicated that they had experienced musculoskeletal pain at work during the past year (American Nurses Association, 2019). In the 2019–2020 HNHN survey, 42% of nurse respondents consider that lifting and repositioning heavy objects, including patients, create a significant level of risk for occupational injuries (ANA, 2020).

Nurses continue to report pain and risk of injury due to patient handling and other tasks. Does availability of and access to safe patient handling and mobility (SPHM) technology translate into healthcare worker use?

No. Eighty-eight percent of respondents in the 2019–2020 HNHN survey either agreed or strongly agreed that they have access to safe patient handling and mobility (SPHM) technology. However, other studies indicate that even if SPHM technology is available, the use of this technology is not consistent due to highly variable SPHM policies and procedures and lack of, or inconsistent management support (Koppelaar et al., 2013; Sampath et al., 2019). Schoenfisch et al.

(2019) found that nursing staff use of available SPHM technology in three acute care settings is limited due to a complex mix of patient, worker, technology, and situational characteristics. Similar results were found by Park et al. (2018) when studying the use of SPHM technology in nursing home settings.

Interestingly, Kayser et al. (2019) found that healthcare consumers in states with SPHM legislation were 60% more likely to have a lift used during their care than healthcare consumers in other states.

This highlights the need for a multifactorial programmatic approach if universal SPHM is to be achieved with the existence of effective and sustainable SPHM programs in all healthcare environments across the care continuum. These standards provide the framework for such an approach.

Universal SPHM has been a goal of ANA for quite some time. Although there is still much to be done before this goal is achieved, ANA continues to work with a broad group of stakeholders including the Veterans Health Administration (VHA), who believe that Universal SPHM is the only way that all professionals who perform high-risk healthcare consumer handling tasks can remain safe in the workplace.

COVID-19 PANDEMIC AND SPHM

The COVID-19 pandemic has had significant impacts particularly on acute and long-term healthcare organizations, workers, and consumers. When extremely large numbers of highly acute and contagious COVID-19 healthcare consumers are present, increased stress is placed on almost every component and program within a healthcare organization. These include healthcare workers, supply chains, the environment of care, and healthcare consumers and their families.

SPHM programs may also be adversely affected by surging COVID-related demands. In the acute care setting, increased demands include proning for acute respiratory distress (ARDS) and physical rehabilitation following extended periods of mechanical ventilation. In the long-term care environment, where extensive handling of healthcare consumers with activities of daily living already occurs multiple times per shift, COVID-related stressors further compromise new demands on staff time, staffing levels, and existing SPHM technology gaps.

Future research may reveal the range of responses to the influences of COVID-19 demands on SPHM programs. Organizations with a strong SPHM program based on consensus standards, such as the ANA SPHM Standards, may be better positioned and adapt more quickly to meet the care and mobility needs of the healthcare consumer in a pandemic. A large nonprofit hospital in Florida, for example, was able to quickly mobilize a SPHM plan for their healthcare consumers and staff. This included placing all dependent healthcare consumers on air-assisted devices regardless of their size and ensuring that a portable or overhead lift and an air-assisted device pump were available in each room. Having SPHM technology readily available in each room allowed the nursing staff to use the technology to reposition smaller/less complex healthcare consumers without help from the facility's injury prevention team, minimizing exposure and preserving personal protective equipment (Labreche, 2020).

Leadership may also influence the responses of SPHM programs to the influences of the pandemic. SPHM managers/coordinators who are experienced or who are certified in SPHM have the expertise necessary to rapidly and successfully respond to the increased demand for healthcare consumer handling and mobilization as well as to effectively participate in organizational decision-making.

THE ESSENTIAL ROLE OF SPHM

As described in these standards, evidence demonstrates that SPHM plays an integral role in the safety and health of healthcare workers, healthcare consumers, and in the wellbeing of healthcare organizations. Well-designed SPHM programs not only reduce the incidence, severity, and costs of healthcare worker injuries associated with manual handling and lifting of healthcare consumers but also reduce healthcare worker turnover and facilitate improved healthcare consumers outcomes (Figure 3).

The need for universal SPHM will only increase as the healthcare consumer population continues to grow and change. SPHM is a critical tool that can be used to facilitate safer care to a healthcare consumer population that is becoming increasingly older, sicker, obese, cognitively impaired, and more dependent on healthcare workers to provide higher levels of assistance (Totzkay, 2018; Waltrip, 2019).

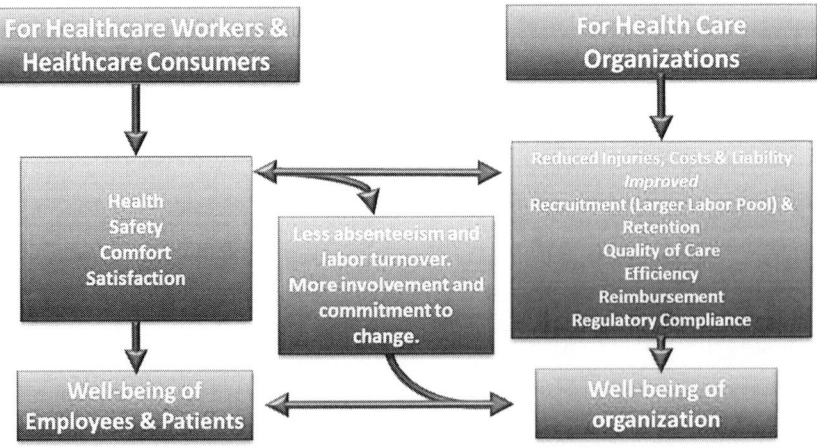

Figure 3. Goals & Benefits of SPHM Programs. Adapted from Enos, 2012; Wilson & Corlett, 2005; Nelson et al., 2008; Occupational Safety and Health Administration (OSHA), 2013a; and OSHA, 2013b.

Over the past decade, there has been a growing awareness that workplace safety is inextricably linked to healthcare consumer safety. As reported by the Institute for Healthcare Improvement (IHI), unless healthcare workers are given the protection, respect, and support they need, they are more likely to make errors, fail to follow safe practices, and not work well in teams (Lucian Leape Institute, 2013).

The COVID-19 pandemic has highlighted the essential need for healthcare organizations and society to maintain the health, safety, and wellbeing of healthcare workers, for safe care to be provided to healthcare consumers.

Unfortunately, healthcare organizations must address tremendous budget shortfalls as a result of the pandemic while addressing a looming healthcare worker shortage and a continued need to improve healthcare consumer outcomes cost-effectively.

Thus, the ANA SPHM standards provide an important framework and guidance for healthcare organizations and workers when addressing these serious issues.

REFERENCES

American Nurses Association. (2019, September). Healthy nurse, healthy nation: Year two highlights 2018–2019. *American Nurse Today, 14*(9). https://www.healthynursehealthynation.org/globalassets/all-images-view-with-media/about/2019-hnhn_highlights.pdf

American Nurses Association. (2020, September). Healthy nurse, healthy nation: Year three highlights 2019–2020. *American Nurse Journal, 14*(9). https://www.healthynursehealthynation.org/globalassets/all-images-view-with-media/about/2020-hnhn_sup-8.pdf

Bureau of Labor Statistics (BLS), Injuries, Illnesses, and Fatalities program. (2020, May). *Fact Sheet: Occupational injuries and illnesses resulting in musculoskeletal disorders (MSDs).* https://www.bls.gov/iif/oshwc/case/msds.htm

Bureau of Labor Statistics (BLS), Survey of Occupational Injuries and Illnesses. (2020, November 4). TABLE R98. Incidence rates for nonfatal occupational injuries and illnesses involving days away from work per 10,000 full-time workers by occupation and selected nature of injury or illness, private industry, 2019. [Data]. https://www.bls.gov/iif/oshwc/osh/case/cd_r98_2019.htm

Bureau of Labor Statistics (BLS), Survey of Occupational Injuries and Illnesses. (2019, November 7). TABLE R98. Incidence rates for nonfatal occupational injuries and illnesses involving days away from work per 10,000 full-time workers by occupation and selected nature of injury or illness, private industry, 2018. [Data]. https://www.bls.gov/iif/oshwc/osh/case/cd_r98_2018.htm

Enos, L. (2012). Evaluating a Safe Patient Handling Program: Beyond Injury Rates. *Proceedings Safe Patient Handling and Mobility Conference 2012.* VISN 8 Patient Safety Center of Inquiry and the Tampa VA Research and Education Foundation.

Kayser, S., Wiggermann, N., & Kumpar, D. (2019). Prevalence of safe patient handling practice in US acute care hospitals. *Proceedings of the Human Factors and Ergonomics Society Annual Meeting, 63,* 1073–1077. https://doi.org/10.1177/1071181319631159

Koppelaar, E., Knibbe, J. J., Miedema, H. S., & Burdorf, A. (2013). The influence of individual and organisational factors on nurses' behaviour to use lifting devices in healthcare. *Applied Ergonomics, 44,* 532–537. https://doi.org/10.1016/j.apergo.2012.11.005

Labreche, M. (2020). Safe patient handling and mobility plan for the COVID-19 units at a level 1 trauma center in Florida. *International Journal of Safe Patient Handling & Mobility, 10*(2), 59–66.

Liberty Mutual Insurance. (2021). Workplace Safety Index 2021: Healthcare and social assistance. 2021_WSI_1003_R2.pdf (libertymutual.com)

Lucian Leape Institute. (2013). *Through the eyes of the workforce: Creating joy, meaning, and safer health care.* The Institute for Healthcare Improvement website: http://www.ihi.org/resources/Pages/Publications/Through-the-Eyes-of-the-Workforce-Creating-Joy-Meaning-and-Safer-Health-Care.aspx

Nelson, A. L. (Ed). (2005). *Safe patient handling and movement: A practical guide for health care professionals.* New York, NY: Springer.

Nelson, A., Collins, J., Siddharthan, K., Matz, M., & Waters, T. (2008). Link between safe patient handling and patient outcomes in Long-Term care. *Rehabilitation Nursing, 33*(1), 33–43.

Occupational Safety and Health Administration. (2013a). *Safe patient handling programs: Effectiveness and cost savings* (OSHA 3729 – 09/2013). https://www.osha.gov/sites/default/files/publications/OSHA3279.pdf

Occupational Safety and Health Administration. (2013b). *Safe patient handling programs: Learn from the leaders.* https://www.osha.gov/sites/default/files/3.6_SPH_profiles_508.pdf

Park, S., Lavender, S. A., Sommerich, C. M., & Patterson, E. S. (2018). Increasing the use of patient lifting devices in nursing homes: Identifying the barriers and facilitators affecting the different adoption stages for an ergonomics intervention. *International Journal of Safe Patient Handling & Mobility, 8,* 9–24.

Sampath, S. L., Wilson, K., Davis, K., & Kotowski, S. (2019). Reality of safe patient handling policies and programs in hospitals across the United States. *International Journal of Safe Patient Handling & Mobility, 9,* 69–76.

Schoenfisch, A. L., Kucera, K. L., Lipscomb, H. J., McIlvaine, J., Becherer, L., James, T., & Avent, S. (2019). Use of assistive devices to lift, transfer, and reposition hospital patients. *Nursing Research, 68,* 3–12. https://doi.org/10.1097/NNR.0000000000000325

Totzkay, D. L. (2018). Multifactorial strategies for sustaining safe patient handling and mobility. *Critical Care Nurse Quarterly, 41,* 340–344. https://doi.org/10.1097/CNQ.0000000000000213

Waltrip, K. (2019). *A survey of healthcare workers on safe patient handling and mobility resource availability, utilization, and adherence* (Doctoral dissertation). https://irl.umsl.edu/dissertation/910

Wilson, J. R. (2005). Chapter 1: A framework and a context for ergonomics methodology. In J. R Wilson, & N. Corlett (Eds.), *Evaluation of human work* (2nd edition; pp. 11). CRC press.

Wilson, J. R., & Corlett, E. N. (Eds.) (1995). *Evaluation of Human Work: A Practical Ergonomics Methodology* (2nd ed.). Taylor & Francis.

Development of the Safe Patient Handling and Mobility Standards

In the summer of 2013, the first version of the *Safe Patient Handling and Mobility: Interprofessional National Standards* was released, followed shortly by the *Implementation Guide to the Safe Patient Handling and Mobility: Interprofessional National Standards*. The Safe Patient Handling and Mobility (SPHM) standards were developed to be:

- Useful in healthcare settings across the continuum of care;

- Useful for healthcare workers, ancillary/support staff, and organizational leadership;

- Realistic and attainable, while raising the bar; and

- Evidence-based and outcome-focused.

The purpose of this revised work was to build on and update the 2013 SPHM Standards and to incorporate up-to-date resources. As much work has been completed in the field of SPHM since the writing of the original Standards, it is imperative to incorporate updated resources and references for the SPHM community.

History of SPHM in the United States

1900–1950s	Various devices developed to move, reposition, and lift patients*
1958	Ted Hoyer developed a hydraulic patient lift*
1972	Journal article indicated nursing staff have higher incidents of back injuries*
1976–1990	Air-assisted patient transfer and movement devices patented*
1984	National Institute for Occupational Safety and Health (NIOSH) recognized lifting injuries in nurses are similar to construction and warehouse workers*
Late 1980s	Overhead lifts and adjustable beds introduced*
1992	*Ergonomic Guidelines for Manual Material Handling* published by State of California, Department of Industrial Relations, Division of Occupational Safety and Health (DOSH) known as CAL/OSHA, and United States, Department of Health and Human Services (DHHS), DHHS (NIOSH) Publication No. 2007-131
Late 1990s	Lift Teams are introduced*
1999	Veterans Health Administration (VHA) Patient Safety Center of Inquiry (PSCI) established first national Safe Patient Handling and Movement Advisory Board
2001	Audrey Nelson, PhD, RN, FAAN, SPHM conducted evidence-based practice research focusing on implementation of SPHM programs and technology
2001	National Collaboration initiated among VHA PSCI, ANA, NIOSH
2001	First Annual SPHM Conference presented by the VHA PSCI and the US Department of Veterans Affairs (VA)
2002	OSHA vs. Beverly Enterprises (US largest nursing home chain) settlement required introduction of lifting technology to avoid ergonomic injuries
2003	*Guidelines for Nursing Homes—Ergonomics for the Prevention of Musculoskeletal Disorders* published by OSHA
2004	ANA's "Handle with Care" Campaign initiated
2005	Texas became the first state to pass a state safe patient handling law. Since that time, 11 other states have passed laws or resolutions related to SPHM
2006	Dr. Audrey Nelson, et al. published a landmark VHA study about necessary components of effective SPHM programs. "Development and evaluation of a multifaceted ergonomics program to prevent injuries associated with patient handling tasks. *Int. J. Nurs. Stud. 43*(6):717–733

2007	Dr. Thomas Waters published the landmark document, "When is it safe to manually lift a patient?" *AJN 107*(8):53–58
2008	National VHA Roll-Out approved by Congress for $205 million for the implementation of SPHM Programs in over 150 health-care systems
2009	Federal Nursing and Healthcare Worker Protection Act introduced in Congress. Reintroduced in 2013 and 2015
2010	First incorporation of SPHM in National Design Guidelines through the work of the Facility Guidelines Institute (FGI). FGI released "Patient Handling and Movement Assessments (PHAMA): A White Paper" to educate design professionals on SPHM
2011	Association of Safe Patient Handling Professionals (ASPHP) established
2011	ASPHP initiated SPHM Professional Certification program. The credentialing organization is now known as the *Certified Safe Patient Handling Professionals*™
2011	The American Journal of SPHM began publication. The journal is now known as the International Journal of SPHM
2012	Joint Commission monograph, "Improving Patient and Worker Safety" published
2012	International Organization for Standardization. Technical report (ISO TR) 12296:2012. *Ergonomics—Manual Handling of People in the Healthcare Sector* published
2013	"SPHM Interprofessional National Standards" published by ANA
2013	OSHA National Emphasis Program (NEP) for programmed inspections of nursing and residential care facilities that included a focus on ergonomics stressors in patient handling and lifting implemented
2014	International Organization for Standardization (ISO) standard 10535:2006. "Hoists for the transfer of disabled persons—requirements and test methods" recognized as a consensus standard by the Food and Drug Administration (FDA)
2015	OSHA Inspection Guidance for Inpatient Healthcare Settings that included a focus on musculoskeletal disorders (MSDs) relating to patient or resident handling issued
2016	Universal SPHM Coalition established jointly by ANA and VHA
2018	*ANA Quality Conference presented value of integrating Fall Prevention, SPHM, and Early Mobility*
2019	"Patient Handling and Movement Assessments", 2nd edition, FGI, published. Added design criteria for bariatrics and facilitating mobilization of healthcare consumers to the original "PHAMA: A White Paper"

| 2020 | First annual ASPHP Educational Conference conducted |
| 2021 | ISO 10535:2021 "Assistive products—Hoists for the transfer of disabled persons—Requirements and test methods" published |

*Used with permission from Guy Fragala (*A History of Safe Patient Handling and Mobility From My Perspective* presentation)

Demographics and Characteristics of the US Population

The population of the United States continues to increase, especially the cohort of older Americans. In December 2020, the US Census Bureau estimated that the median age reached a new maximum of 38.4, due in large part to the aging baby boomer category (US Census Bureau, 2020). Life expectancy also continued to increase after several years of decline, reaching 78.7 years in 2018 (Centers for Disease Control, National Center for Health Statistics, 2020a). Organizations and manufacturers are responding by expanding SPHM programs and technologies into additional healthcare environments including long-term care, home care, emergency response, and ambulatory settings.

Obesity rates continue to rise steadily in all 50 states (CDC NCHS, 2020b). Each state has now recorded an obesity rate of at least 20%. From 2000 through 2018, the prevalence of obesity rose from 30.5% to 42.4%, with the category of severe obesity (BMI > 40) growing from 4.7% to 9.2%. Factors including race, socioeconomic status, and age influence obesity rates. This situation presents one of the highest risks and stressors for healthcare workers.

Morbidity rates affect inpatient hospitalization, healthcare consumer characteristics, and the need for SPHM. In 2020, the CDC reported that the 10 leading causes of death in 2018 remain unchanged from 2017 (CDC NCHS, 2020a). The leading causes (from highest to lowest) were heart disease, cancer, unintentional injuries, lower respiratory disease, stroke, Alzheimer's disease, diabetes, influenza and pneumonia, kidney disease, and suicide. Some of these conditions require extended inpatient care, presenting increased risks from immobility, and an increased need for healthcare consumer handling and rehabilitation. Others require increased care outside the hospital environment, further highlighting the need to expand SPHM to these settings.

REFERENCES

CDC National Center for Health Statistics. (2020a). *Mortality in the United States, 2018* (NCHS Data Brief No. 355). https://www.cdc.gov/nchs/products/databriefs/db355.htm

CDC National Center for Health Statistics. (2020b). *Prevalence of obesity and severe obesity among adults: United States, 2017–2018* (NCHS Data Brief No. 360). https://www.cdc.gov/nchs/products/databriefs/db360.htm

US Census Bureau. (2020, December 15). *Census bureau releases 2020 demographic analysis estimates* [Press release]. https://www.census.gov/newsroom/press-releases/2020/2020-demographic-analysis-estimates.html

Safe Patient Handling and Mobility Trends and Issues

1. FACILITATING AN EFFECTIVE CULTURE OF SAFETY

According to The Joint Commission (TJC), the definition of Safety Culture is the sum of what an organization does in the pursuit of safety. TJC further explains safety culture as "the product of individual and group beliefs, values, attitudes, perceptions, competencies and patterns of behavior that determine the organization's commitment to quality and patient safety" (The Joint Commission, 2017). To achieve this culture requires a continuum of care approach with commitment, collaboration, and communication at all levels of the organization, e.g., leaders, managers, and employees.

Health care organizations often use the principles of a "just culture" to establish a culture of safety. Such organizations strive to avoid a punitive environment where employees are solely blamed for errors. Instead, they design reliable systems with embedded barriers to prevent human error and reduce the likelihood of severe or fatal errors. Human behavior is managed within the systems, and everyone is encouraged to communicate safety risks, hazards, and system flaws.

James Reason describes a "just culture" as one in which "people are encouraged, even rewarded, for providing essential, safety-related information; but clear lines are drawn between human error and at-risk or reckless behaviors" (Reason, p. 195). He also elaborates on the meanings of a "reporting culture," as one in which people are confident in reporting their errors and near-misses (Reason, 1997).

A foundational element in a culture of safety is the ethical responsibility of all registered nurses (and other healthcare workers) to protect the health and safety of healthcare consumers and themselves (ANA, 2009). This can be supported through systems designed to recognize and educate on the three distinct types of human responses during critical interactions: inadvertent slips or lapse (human errors), risk not recognized or believed (at-risk behavior), and conscious disregard of unreasonable risk (reckless behavior; Paradiso & Sweeney, 2019).

Many health care organizations are also utilizing the elements of "high reliability" to achieve a culture of safety. Other complex, hazardous systems such as airline, nuclear power, and oil industries have implemented high reliability principles to elevate safety as a core value and reduce errors. Key principles include an openness to continuous improvement and change, a preoccupation with failure, a reluctance to simplify, and a sensitivity to operations, among others (Hales & Chakravorty, 2016).

Using a collaborative approach, within a culture of safety, enables all healthcare workers to provide valuable input and feedback to develop safe, effective SPHM programs.

REFERENCES

American Nurses Association. (2009). *Patient safety: Rights of registered nurses when considering a patient assignment.* https://www.nursingworld.org/practice-policy/nursing-excellence/official-position-statements/id/patient-safety-rights-of-registered-nurses-when-considering-a-patient-assignment/

Hales, D. N., & Chakravorty, S. S. (2016). Creating high reliability organizations using mindfulness. *Journal of Business Research, 69,* 2873–2881. https://doi.org/10.1016/j.jbusres.2015.12.056

The Joint Commission. (2017, March 1). The essential role of leadership in developing a safety culture. *Sentinel Event Alert* (57). https://www.jointcommission.org/-/media/tjc/documents/resources/patient-safety-topics/sentinel-event/sea_57_safety_culture_leadership_0317pdf.pdf

Paradiso, L., & Sweeney, N. (2019). Just culture: It's more than policy. *Nursing Management, 50*(6), 38–45. https://journals.lww.com/nursingmanagement/Fulltext/2019/06000/Just_culture__It_s_more_than_policy.9.aspx

Reason, J. (1997). *Managing the Risks of Organizational Accidents.* Ashgate.

2. FOCUSING ON HEALTHCARE CONSUMER OUTCOMES

The body of evidence that supports the role of safe patient handling and mobility (SPHM) to facilitate positive healthcare consumer outcomes has continued to grow since the publication of the first ANA SPHM Interprofessional National Standards.

Gibson, Costa, and Sampson (2017) conducted a systematic review of studies that examined the association between healthcare worker health and safety and healthcare consumer outcomes. They reported several key findings to support the positive impact of SPHM programs on healthcare worker musculoskeletal health and on healthcare consumer outcomes.

The most significant impact of SPHM on healthcare consumer outcomes appears to be as the facilitator of early and progressive mobilization, which encompasses a continuum of activities from in-bed mobilization to supervised ambulation.

It is well documented that insufficient physical mobility during hospitalization and the associated series of cascading and functional decline-related problems result in serious consequences for healthcare consumers and healthcare organizations (Smart et al., 2018).

Early mobility programs are widely promoted in acute care settings and have demonstrated reduction in complications related to immobility, such as pneumonia, pressure ulcers, delirium, falls, longer length of stay, complex hospital-to-home transitions, and death (Hoyer et al., 2016; LaVigne & Arnold, 2016). Increased early mobilization not only positively affects healthcare consumers' physical functioning but also their emotional and social well-being leading to enhanced comfort, satisfaction, and quality of life (Kalisch et al., 2014). In long-term care, mobility programs play an equally important role aimed at restoring or maintaining mobility and functional independence of residents for as long as possible.

Although there is need for more research to demonstrate the impact of specific SPHM-related interventions on early mobility, an evidence-based multifaceted SPHM programmatic approach can be integrated with recognized requirements of early mobility programs to protect healthcare workers and healthcare consumers from harm (Wyatt et al., 2020).

Gibson et al. (2017) reported that SPHM programs and policies and procedures around use of mechanical lifting devices can improve healthcare consumer mobility outcomes by up to 12%, and Basset et al. (2012) reported that a lack of overhead lifts is identified as a barrier to early mobilization.

Klein et al. (2015) reported that the use of bed features, a mobile lift, and assistance from the rehabilitation and lift teams enabled successful progression of healthcare consumers' levels of mobility in a neurologic ICU.

Darragh et al. (2013) reported that there is evidence that the use of SPHM technology during rehabilitation has therapeutic applications especially for medically complex and for bariatric healthcare consumers. Within the context of using SPHM to mobilize healthcare consumers to reduce the risk of adverse hospital-acquired harm, there is evidence to support that the use of SPHM technology and related policies and procedures can reduce the risk of healthcare facility-acquired pressure injuries up to 17% (Gibson et al., 2017).

One hospital reported a 43% decrease in hospital-acquired pressure ulcers (Walden et al., 2013) after implementing SPHM programs, and another reported a 50% decrease in stages III and IV hospital-acquired pressure ulcers during the first year after SPHM program implementation (Kennedy & Kopp, 2015).

To further support the importance of SPHM in preventing pressure injuries, wound care organizations around the world advise the use of friction-reducing sheets or lift technology to reposition or transfer healthcare consumers in bed to avoid such injuries (Agency for Healthcare Research and Quality, 2011; Australian Wound Management Association, 2012; Brienza et al., 2015; European Pressure Ulcer Advisory Panel, 2014).

A reduction in healthcare consumer fall rates has been reported following implementation of SPHM programs and use of technology such as overhead lifts (The Joint Commission, 2012; Kennedy & Kopp, 2015; Spritzer et al., 2015).

SPHM is considered "a critical element of universal fall precaution and especially important for healthcare consumers who require assistance with transfers" by the Agency for Health Care Research and Quality (AHRQ, 2013).

In long-term care, multifaceted SPHM programs that included the use of sit-to-stand devices were reported to decrease rates of pressure injuries and falls in four facilities (Gucer et al., 2013).

Similarly, another study in a long-term care setting, found that using SPHM technology and practices also lowered fall risk among residents and increased their physical functioning and activity level, improved urinary continence, lowered levels of depression, and improved alertness during the day (Nelson et al., 2008).

Being lifted and moved manually can be a painful and undignified experience for healthcare consumers and can cause soft tissue injury. This contributes to a negative healthcare consumer experience. The use of mechanical lifting devices and positioning devices have been shown to improve healthcare consumer comfort and safety (Gibson et al., 2017).

Although not well researched, SPHM may also play an important role in mitigating missed nursing care in relation to healthcare consumer mobilization in both acute and long-term care settings. Missed nursing care is defined as any aspect of required healthcare consumer care that is omitted (either in part or in whole) or significantly delayed by nursing staff. Missed care or rationing of care is associated with increased adverse healthcare consumer safety events, and a higher likelihood of healthcare consumer death (Hessels et al., 2019). Missed nursing care occurs for various reasons, including accessibility of staff and material resources to assist in healthcare consumer care activities, work environment values including organizational and unit culture, and dysfunctional teamwork (Agency for Healthcare Research and Quality, 2019).

Two healthcare consumer care tasks that nurses most frequently do not complete as planned are ambulating and repositioning, leading to the negative consequences of immobility that were previously noted (Hessels et al., 2019; Kalisch & Xie, 2014).

Although the causative factors for missed nursing care may be multiple and interrelated, it is feasible that a well-designed multifaceted SPHM program that includes standardized SPHM healthcare consumer assessments for mobility, sufficient quantity of appropriate and readily accessible SPHM technology, and competency-based staff training on technology use, may help reduce the incidence of missed repositioning and ambulation activities, and related implications for a health care organization.

The evidence, thus far, indicates that where SPHM intersects with the multiple protocols and tasks required to promote safe and early mobility of healthcare consumers, it plays a key role to facilitate holistic healthcare consumer care and the associated benefits to healthcare organizations.

WORKPLACE VIOLENCE AND SPHM

Violence by healthcare consumers against healthcare workers has increased significantly over the past decade with serious and sometimes deadly consequences for workers (Bureau of Labor Statistics, 2020).

Close physical contact between healthcare consumers and healthcare workers that occurs during manual handling tasks may initiate violent episodes especially with healthcare consumers who are cognitively impaired. Consistent use of SPHM technology, such as ceiling and floor-based lifts, appears to reduce the risk of healthcare consumer-initiated violence (Collins et al., 2006; Pihl-Thingvad et al., 2018; Risør et al., 2017).

In a study that evaluated a large nursing home corporation's Safe Resident Handling Program (SRHP) over a period of 10 years (2006–2016), researchers found that besides a decrease in the rates of musculoskeletal disorders associated with manual resident handling, worker claims for "aggression" injuries were reduced by about 12% following the SRHP and for at least 6 years afterward (Kurowski & El Ghaziri, 2019).

REFERENCES

Agency for Healthcare Research and Quality. (2011). *Preventing pressure ulcers in hospitals: A toolkit for improving quality of care.* https://www.ahrq.gov/sites/default/files/publications/files/putoolkit.pdf

Agency for Healthcare Research and Quality. (2013). *Preventing falls in hospitals: A toolkit for improving quality of care.* (AHRQ Publication No. 13-0015-EF 2013). https://www.ahrq.gov/patient-safety/settings/hospital/fall-prevention/toolkit/index.html

Agency for Healthcare Research and Quality, Patient Safety Network. (2019, Sept. 7). Missed Patient safety 101 primer: Missed nursing care. https://psnet.ahrq.gov/primer/missed-nursing-care

Australian Wound Management Association. (2012). *Pan Pacific clinical practice guideline for the prevention and management of pressure injury.* Osborne Park, WA: Cambridge Media.

Bassett, R. D., Vollman, K. M., Brandwene, L., & Murray, T. (2012). Integrating a multidisciplinary mobility programme into intensive care practice (IMMPTP): A multicentre collaborative. *Intensive and Critical Care Nursing, 28,* 88–97. https://doi.org/10.1016/j.iccn.2011.12.001

Brienza, D., Deppisch, M., Gillespie, C., Goldberg, M., Gruccio, P., Jordan, R., Lachenbruch, C., Logan, S., Mackey, D., Sylvia, C., & Thurman, K. (2015). *Do lift slings significantly change the efficacy of therapeutic support surfaces?* National Pressure Ulcer Advisory Panel website: 1a._npuap-lift-sling-white-p. pdf (ymaws.com)

Bureau of Labor Statistics. (2020, April). *Fact sheet: Workplace violence in healthcare, 2018.* https://www.bls.gov/iif/oshwc/cfoi/workplace-violence-healthcare-2018.htm

Collins, J. W., Nelson, A., & Sublet, V. (2006). *Safe lifting and movement of nursing home residents.* (DHHS [NIOSH] Publication No. 2006-117). Cincinnati, OH: National Institute for Occupational Safety and Health. Centers for Disease Control and Prevention, National Institute for Occupational Safety and Health website: http://www.cdc.gov/niosh/docs/2006-117/

Darragh, A. R., Campo, M. A., Frost, L., Miller, M., Pentico, M., & Margulis, H. (2013). Safe-patient-handling equipment in therapy practice: Implications for rehabilitation. *American Journal of Occupational Therapy, 67,* 45–53. https://doi.org/10.5014/ajot.2013.005389

European Pressure Ulcer Advisory Panel. (2014). NPUAP-EPUAP-PPPIA Pressure Ulcer Treatment & Prevention. 2014 Quick Reference Guide. quick-reference-guide-digital-npuap-epuap-pppia-jan2016.pdf

Gibson, K., Costa, B., & Sampson, A. (2017). *Linking worker health and safety with patient outcomes: A systematic review.* Institute of Safety, Compensation and Recovery Research website: http://www.iscrr.com.au/__data/assets/pdf_file/0006/1321719/Evidence-Review_Linking-worker-health-and-safety-with-patient-outcomes.pdf

Gucer, P. W., Gaitens, J., Oliver, M., & McDiarmid, M. A. (2013). Sit-stand powered mechanical lifts in long-term care and resident quality indicators. *Journal of Occupational and Environmental Medicine, 55,* 36–44. https://doi.org/10.1097/JOM.0b013e3182749c35

Hessels, A. J., Paliwal, M., Weaver, S. H., Siddiqui, D., & Wurmser, T. A. (2019). Impact of patient safety culture on missed nursing care and adverse patient events. *Journal of Nursing Care Quality, 34,* 287–294. https://doi.org/10.1097/NCQ.0000000000000378

Hoyer, E. H., Friedman, M., Lavezza, A., Wagner-Kosmakos, K., Lewis-Cherry, R., Skolnik, J. L., & Needham, D. M. (2016). Promoting mobility and reducing length of stay in hospitalized general medicine patients: A quality-improvement project. *Journal of Hospital* Medicine, *11,* 341–347. https://doi.org/10.1002/jhm.2546

The Joint Commission. (2012). *Improving patient and worker safety: Opportunities for synergy, collaboration and innovation.* http://www.jointcommission.org/assets/1/18/TJC-ImprovingPatientAndWorkerSafety-Monograph.pdf

Kalisch, B. J., & Xie, B. (2014). Errors of omission: Missed nursing care. *Western Journal of Nursing Research, 36,* 875–890. https://doi.org/10.1177/0193945914531859

Kalisch, B. J., Lee, S., & Dabney, B. W. (2014). Outcomes of inpatient mobilization: A literature review. *Journal of Clinical Nursing, 23,* 1486–1501. https://doi.org/10.1111/jocn.12315

Kennedy, B., & Kopp, T. (2015). Safe patient handling protects employees too. *Nursing, 45*(8), 65–7. https://doi.org/10.1097/01.NURSE.0000466460.70493.55

Klein, K., Mulkey, M., Bena, J. F., & Albert, N. M. (2015). Clinical and psychological effects of early mobilization in patients treated in a neurologic ICU: A comparative study. *Critical Care Medicine, 43,* 865–873. https://doi.org/10.1097/CCM.0000000000000787

Kurowski, A., & El Ghaziri, M. (2019). The role of safe handling and mobilization in reducing type II workplace violence in healthcare settings (CPH News and Views, Issue 62). The UMass Lowell, Center for the Promotion of Health in the New England Workplace website: https://www.uml.edu/Research/CPH-NEW/News/emerging-topics/News-views-62.aspx

LaVigne, A., & Arnold, M. (2016). Decision making for safe patient handling and mobility technology in an early mobility program: A case report. *International Journal of Safe Patient Handling & Movement, 6,* 65–72.

Nelson, A. L., Collins, J., Siddharthan, K., Matz, M., & Waters, T. (2008). Link between safe patient handling and patient outcomes in longterm care. *Rehabilitation Nursing, 33*(1), 33–43. Study - Link Between Safe Patient Handling and Patient Outcomes in LongTerm Care (iprsmediquipe.com)

Pihl-Thingvad, J., Brandt, L. P. A., & Andersen, L. L. (2018). Consistent use of assistive devices for patient transfer is associated with less patient-initiated violence: Cross-sectional study among health care workers at general hospitals. *Workplace Health & Safety, 66,* 453–461. https://doi.org/10.1177/2165079917752714

Risør, B. W., Casper, S. D., Andersen, L. L., & Sørensen, J. (2017). A multi-component patient-handling intervention improves attitudes and behaviors for safe patient handling and reduces aggression experienced by nursing staff: A controlled before-after study. *Applied Ergonomics, 60*, 74–82. https://doi.org/10.1016/j.apergo.2016.10.011

Smart, D. A., Dermody, G., Coronado, M. E., & Wilson, M. (2018). Mobility programs for the hospitalized older adult: A scoping review. *Gerontology and Geriatric Medicine, 4*:2333721418808146. https://doi.org/10.1177/2333721418808146

Spritzer, S. D., Riordan, K. C., Berry, J., Corbett, B. M., Gerke, J. K., Hoerth, M. T., Crepeau, A. Z., Drazkowski, J. F., Sirven, J. I., & Noe, K. H. (2015). Fall prevention and bathroom safety in the epilepsy monitoring unit. *Epilepsy & Behavior, 48*, 75–78. https://doi.org/10.1016/j.yebeh.2015.05.026

Walden, C. M., Bankard, S. B., Cayer, B., Floyd, W. B., Garrison, H. G., Hickey, T., Holfer, L. D., Rotondo, M. F., & Pories, W. J. (2013). Mobilization of the obese patient and prevention of injury. *Annals of Surgery, 258*, 646–50; discussion 650–1. https://doi.org/10.1097/SLA.0b013e3182a5039f

Wyatt, S., Meacci, K., & Arnold, M. (2020). Integrating safe patient handling and early mobility: Combining quality initiatives. *Journal of Nursing Care Quality, 35*, 130–134. https://doi.org/10.1097/NCQ.0000000000000425

3. IMPROVEMENTS IN SAFE PATIENT HANDLING AND MOBILITY TECHNOLOGY

Innovations in safe patient handling and mobility (SPHM) technology continue in response to an increased demand for ways to safely mobilize healthcare consumers. As manufacturers research the needs across the continuum of care, they are designing new devices, which can assist with a single task, such as turning; and those designed to assist with multiple tasks, such as ambulation and lifting. A wider range of devices with increased weight capacities is also available to accommodate individuals of size (bariatric; Matz et al., 2019).

Notably, some manufacturers are providing evidence for their devices related to the effects on quality of healthcare consumer care as well as the healthcare worker injury risk reduction. Many manufacturers also solicit input from healthcare workers about their experience with SPHM technology and for suggested technology improvements to enhance safety and better meet healthcare consumer needs.

Quantifiable data on the reduction of risk assist buyers in justifying purchases and comparing similar products in a device category. These data help promote increased acceptance of SPHM technology utilization by all clinical disciplines.

Improvements designed to enhance the operation and movement of both floor and overhead lifts continue to be made. Examples include equipment interfaces that enable the user to operate the controls more easily, access instructions, and capture usage data. Power-assist mobile lifts can be purchased that have motorized drives to propel the devices in multiple directions, turn the wheels, and move the healthcare consumer, thus reducing exertion for the healthcare worker (Matz et al., 2019). Portable total and sit-to-stand lifts are being designed to allow for more functional activity and can be adjusted to provide different levels of support as the healthcare consumer progresses through rehabilitation (Matz et al., 2019). Powered spreader bars are options that enable the healthcare worker to change more easily the position of the healthcare consumer from reclining to sitting.

An increasing number of slings are available for use with existing overhead lifts that enable progressive mobility during rehabilitation. New overhead lift motors can be recessed in the track, and some have blocks/stops, which facilitate stable rehabilitation exercises (Matz et al., 2019).

Electronic beds have additional features to assist not only with turning but with sitting, standing, and egress.

REFERENCE

Matz, M., Celona, J., Martin, M., McCoskey, K., & Nelson, G. G. (2019). *Patient handling and mobility assessments*. (2nd ed.). The Facility Guidelines Institute website: https://www.fgiguidelines.org/wp-content/uploads/2019/10/FGI-Patient-Handling-and-Mobility-Assessments_191008.pdf

4. THE FUTURE OF SAFE PATIENT HANDLING AND MOBILITY TECHNOLOGY

Healthcare has seen a significant advance in the use of robotics and artificial intelligence (AI) during the past decade. In several countries around the world, governments are heavily investing in the development of AI-enabled robotic-assistive devices. Some devices for home use can move healthcare consumers and complete simple care tasks and health monitoring. The goal of this growing movement is to address the mobility and care needs of an expanding aging population, insufficient number of healthcare workers, and provision of community-based care that reduces the need for hospitalization whenever possible (Kajitani & Wakita, 2017; Litwin, 2020; Van Aerschot & Parviainen, 2020).

AI technology is also increasingly incorporated into the design of powered safe patient handling and mobility (SPHM) devices such as floor and overhead lifts. These features improve device safety for healthcare workers and healthcare consumers. Examples include powered steering or movement, object proximity controls, intuitive control interfaces, and a more comprehensive ability to collect data about device use, and maintenance needs. These and many other features allow customization of device functions to suit a healthcare consumer's clinical and mobility needs (Matz et al., 2019; Sivakanthan et al., 2021). Automated lift systems that allow a healthcare consumer to transfer to and from a wheelchair to a bed using a computer-based application that is operated by the healthcare worker are available, as are robotic-assist transfer systems that can be operated by the healthcare consumer without healthcare worker assistance. Although these systems may currently be cost prohibitive for many healthcare consumers, the increased use and advances in robotic technology should make these technologies more affordable and practical for community use in the not too distant future (Humphreys et al., 2017; Sivakanthan et al., 2021).

Research into the use of exoskeletal technology is also increasing, both in the application of healthcare consumer handling and in the operating room environment for use by surgeons to reduce upper extremity fatigue during surgery. Exoskeletons worn by healthcare consumers are showing promise as a rehabilitation tool to promote mobility for healthcare consumers with gait-related disorders (Cha et al., 2020; Young & Ferris, 2016).

Previously, exoskeletal technology has mostly been used in the military and manufacturing environments to enhance the physical capabilities of soldiers and workers to perform physically demanding tasks such as manual material handling. Limitations of exoskeleton use, such as the need to custom fit the device for each individual worker, have to be addressed if they are to be considered as another tool to reduce healthcare worker injuries related to healthcare consumer handling. Healthcare consumer safety and experience must also be evaluated when considering the use of exoskeleton technology by healthcare workers (Robertson et al., 2020; Turja et al., 2020; Zheng, 2020).

As the use of robotic and AI technology grows in the SPHM and rehabilitation industry, there is also a global effort to harmonize medical device regulations/

standards. The goals of harmonization include reducing the time to bring newer technologies to market and enhancing healthcare consumer and healthcare worker safety. The International Organization for Standardization's (ISO) 10535:2021 "Hoists for the transfer of disabled persons—requirements and test methods" is one of the global standards that United States-based manufacturers and distributors of powered lifts and slings are expected to meet. This recently revised standard specifically addresses the increased use of AI in lift technology and compatibility-related issues due to the wide-ranging variability in design of healthcare consumer lifts and slings. The goal of this standard is to increase healthcare consumer safety and comfort by decreasing the risk of healthcare worker error when choosing and using SPHM technology.

The use of SPHM technology has been shown to be beneficial in preventing healthcare worker injuries and facilitating improved healthcare consumer outcomes in the hospital and long-term care settings. However, there is still a need for SPHM technology that is designed to work well in settings with specific healthcare consumer populations and/or work environments, such as behavioral health, emergency services, the operating room, and home health.

The COVID-19 pandemic has accelerated the changes that were already occurring in US healthcare delivery models prior to 2020. These changes included a dramatic increase in the use of telemedicine to deliver care (Koonin et al., 2020) and a significant increase in the "hospital at home" model of care (American Association of Medical Colleges, 2020). It is expected that the use of these care models will continue to expand after the pandemic is over because of the valuable benefits that have been demonstrated when care is provided in the home setting. These benefits include increased access to care especially in underserved communities, improved mortality rates, reduced hospital readmissions, and costs.

An important facilitator in providing successful home-based care will be access to SPHM technology that is designed to be functional for the home care setting and that can be easily used by healthcare consumers, family members, and others providing care. The benefits of SPHM to facilitate and maintain healthcare consumer care and mobility that have been reported in the acute care setting can be realized for the home care healthcare consumer population.

It will be critical that the SPHM technology of the future is not only easy to use for healthcare workers but also that it is integrated within a system of care to facilitate improved outcomes for healthcare consumers. Such outcomes include pressure injury and fall prevention, and improvements in mobilization, and rehabilitation. Finally, and importantly, SPHM technology must interface seamlessly with the care environment in which it is to be used.

REFERENCES

American Association of Medical Colleges. (2020, Sept. 29). Interest in hospital-at-home programs explodes during COVID-19. https://www.aamc.org/news-insights/interest-hospital-home-programs-explodes-during-covid-19

Cha, J. S., Monfared, S., Stefanidis, D., Nussbaum, M. A., & Yu, D. (2020). Supporting surgical teams: Identifying needs and barriers for exoskeleton implementation in the operating room. *Human Factors, 62*, 377–390. https://doi.org/10.1177/0018720819879271

Humphreys, H. C., Choi, Y. M., & Book, W. J. (2017). Advanced patient transfer assist device with intuitive interaction control. *Assistive Technology*, 1–11. https://doi.org/10.1080/10400435.2017.1396564

International Organization for Standardization. (2006). *Hoists for the Transfer of Disabled Persons—Requirements and Test Methods* (ISO 10535:2021). Geneva, Switzerland.

Kajitani, I., & Wakita, Y. (2017). An introduction to the development of transfer assistive robots in Japan. *Studies in Health Technology and Informatics, 242*, 465–471.

Koonin, L. M., Hoots, B., Tsang, C. A., Leroy, Z., Farris, K., Tilman Jolly, B., Antall, P., McCabe, B, Zelis, C. B. R., Tong, I., & Harris, A. M. (2020, October 30). Trends in the use of telehealth during the emergence of the COVID-19 pandemic—United States, January–March 2020. *Morbidity and Mortality Weekly Report, 69*, 1595–1599. https://doi.org/10.15585/mmwr.mm6943a3

Litwin, A. S. (2020). *Technological change in health care delivery: Its drivers and consequences for work and workers*. Berkeley: UC Berkeley Labor Center. The UC Berkeley Labor Center website: https://laborcenter.berkeley.edu/wp-content/uploads/2020/07/Technological-Change-in-Health-Care-Delivery.pdf

Matz, M., Celona, J., Martin, M., McCoskey, K., & Nelson, G. G. (2019). *Patient handling and mobility assessments*. (2nd ed.). The Facility Guidelines Institute website: https://www.fgiguidelines.org/wp-content/uploads/2019/10/FGI-Patient-Handling-and-Mobility-Assessments_191008.pdf

Robertson, L.D., Syron, L., Flynn, M., Teske, T., Hsiao, H., Lu, J., & Lowe, B. (2020). Exoskeletons and occupational health equity. https://blogs.cdc.gov/niosh-science-blog/2020/12/14/exoskeletons-health-equity/

Sivakanthan, S., Blaauw, E., Greenhalgh, M., Koontz, A. M., Vegter, R., & Cooper, R. A. (2021). Person transfer assist systems: A literature review. *Disability and Rehabilitation: Assistive Technology, 16*, 270–279. https://doi.org/10.1080/17483107.2019.1673833

Turja, T., Saurio, R., Katila, J., Hennala, L., Pekkarinen, S., & Melkas, H. (2020). Intention to use exoskeletons in geriatric care work: Need for ergonomic and social design. *Ergonomics in Design*, 1064804620961577. https://doi.org/10.1177/1064804620961577

Van Aerschot, L., & Parviainen, J. (2020). Robots responding to care needs? A multitasking care robot pursued for 25 years, available products offer simple entertainment and instrumental assistance. *Ethics and Information Technology*, 22, 247–256. https://doi.org/10.1007/s10676-020-09536-0

Young, A. J., & Ferris, D. P. (2016). State of the art and future directions for lower limb robotic exoskeletons. *IEEE Transactions on Neural Systems and Rehabilitation Engineering*, 25, 171–182. https://doi.org/10.1109/TNSRE.2016.2521160

Zheng, L. (2020, November 4). Can exoskeletons reduce musculoskeletal disorders in healthcare workers? The Centers for Disease Control and Prevention, NIOSH Science Blog: https://blogs.cdc.gov/niosh-science-blog/2020/11/04/exoskeletons-hc/

5. INCLUDING SAFE PATIENT HANDLING AND MOBILITY IN DESIGN AND CONSTRUCTION

Manual handling, moving, and mobilizing healthcare consumers is hazardous work. In recognition of this fact, in 2010, the Facility Guideline Institute (FGI) developed and approved safe patient handling and mobility (SPHM) design requirements for their *Guidelines for Design and Construction of Health Care Facilities*. The goal of these design requirements was to support safe patient handling and movement practices. The need to educate design professionals on safe patient handling, movement, and mobility (SPHM) was apparent, so the FGI committee wrote the original Patient Handling and Mobility (PHAMA) White Paper to provide information about the rationale for, and relationship of, the physical environment with safe patient handling techniques. Continuing and expanding on the original goal, the FGI published the second edition of *Patient Handling and Movement Assessments* in 2019 (Matz et al., 2019). The second edition updates information on design requirements and incorporates those for care of individuals of size and to facilitate healthcare consumer mobilization. The second edition also provides detailed information to facilitate and implement SPHM programs as well as to develop a business plan to assist organizations in ensuring appropriate technology and program elements are included for success. States that adopt these *Guidelines* are required, unless an exception is made, to follow design criteria within, including the PHAMA. The Joint Commission has no specific criteria statements related to SPHM, but it does require facilities that are building new edifices or undergoing major renovations to use the FGI *Guidelines*, or the state construction guidelines, which are often FGI *Guidelines*. Since the FGI *Guidelines* include the PHAMA, such construction should abide by the PHAMA.

The Safety Risk Assessment (SRA) is a tool to assist organizations and design professionals with incorporating design practices that reduce common risks found in healthcare environments. The SRA targets six areas of safety (patient handling, infections, falls, medication errors, security, and injuries of behavioral health) as required in the Facility Guidelines Institute (FGI) design and construction guidelines. The SRA uses a proactive approach to safety in healthcare facility design, and, in doing so, identifies potentially unsafe conditions of the built environment. It provides discussion prompts for a multidisciplinary team and an evidence-based design (EBD) approach to identify solutions to risks. The tool has maximum potential early in the design process, using systems thinking, and a multidisciplinary approach. Anyone (design team, healthcare organization, and risk management team) can lead the process, but all stakeholders need to be at the table (Center for Health Design, 2017).

REFERENCES

Center for Health Design. (2014, 2017). *Safety risk assessment toolkit: A process to mitigate risk (CHD Tools)*. The Center for Health Design website: https://www.healthdesign.org/sra

Matz, M., Celona, J., Martin, M., McCoskey, K., & Nelson, G. G. (2019). *Patient handling and mobility assessments*. (2nd ed.). The Facilities Guidelines Institute website: https://www.fgiguidelines.org/wp-content/uploads/2019/10/FGI-Patient-Handling-and-Mobility-Assessments_191008.pdf

6. BUILDING AND SUSTAINING THE BUSINESS CASE

Implementation of a multifaceted safe patient handling and mobility (SPHM) program, as described in these standards, has been shown to decrease healthcare worker injuries and associated workers' compensation costs and produce a return on investment (ROI) ranging from 2 to 4 years (Matz et al., 2019; Teeple et al., 2017). However, the value and ROI are far greater than solely reducing the direct costs of healthcare worker musculoskeletal disorders (MSDs). Evidence supports the positive relationship of SPHM as a facilitator of early and safe mobility of healthcare consumers, reducing the negative outcomes of immobility. Other benefits include reductions in healthcare consumer falls and improved healthcare consumer experience, as well as improved healthcare worker efficiency and perceived improvements in safety culture (Gibson et al., 2017; Matz et al., 2019; Occupational Safety and Health Administration, 2016).

There is a growing body of evidence to support that the same characteristics of the healthcare work environment that contribute to physical injuries and psychological harm to healthcare workers, such as MSDs, workplace violence, fatigue, stress, and burnout, also contribute to adverse events for healthcare consumers. These factors negatively impact an organization by increasing the cost of healthcare worker injuries and staff turnover, decreasing reimbursement for "never" events such as falls, and contributing to sub-optimal healthcare consumer experience metrics (Berkowitz, 2016; Gibson et al., 2017; Loeppke et al., 2017).

As many healthcare organizations in the United States now face considerable financial challenges as a result of the COVID-19 pandemic, it is more important than ever to demonstrate the ROI of SPHM using a system approach that underscores the relationship between the benefits to healthcare workers, healthcare consumers, and the organization. Organizations must understand that such programs improve organizational effectiveness while enhancing healthcare consumer safety and outcomes and supporting healthier workforces (Loeppke et al., 2016).

Periodic benchmarking and recalculation of ROI are necessary to sustain and expand a SPHM program and demonstrate its performance. Establishing an organization's baseline employee injury and healthcare consumer safety statistics and demonstrating program outcome trends over time are critical steps in communicating SPHM program performance for continued support and expansion.

Employee benchmarking data can often be obtained through the risk management/workers compensation provider. Many have aggregate databases that can be useful in highlighting average costs and other statistics for organizations similar in size and composition.

For example, a 2016 report from Aon indicated that for healthcare systems implementing the ANA SPHM Interprofessional National Standards, the average total cost of a workers' compensation claim was reduced by 23% ($6,000 versus $7,800) compared with systems not using the standards. The data included historical claim information of $2.4 billion incurred loss dollars from all 50 states, from 2005 through 2016.

Repeating the analysis in 2018, Aon found increased validation for implementing the standards. In a larger dataset of $3.0 billion incurred loss dollars, the average total cost of a workers' compensation claim was 36% lower per cost claim ($5,900 versus $9,200) for healthcare systems using the standards. The evidence from the 2016 and 2018 reports shows that the standards may be a positive influence on the overall culture of safety and an effective cost mitigation strategy. See Table 1 for more details.

Table 1. Comparison of average total cost of a worker's compensation claims for healthcare systems following or not following the SPHM Interprofessional National Standards.

Data Analyzed	2016		2018	
	Following SPHM Standards	**Not Following** SPHM Standards	**Following or Partially Following** SPHM Standards	**Not Following** SPHM Standards
Average total cost of a worker's compensation claim	$6,000	$7,800	$5,900	$9,200
% Reduction	23%		36%	

Reprinted from "Aon health care workers compensation barometer," *by V. Jones et al. (2018)*. Copyright 2018 by Aon.

REFERENCES

Berkowitz, B. (2016). The patient experience and patient satisfaction: Measurement of a complex dynamic. *Online Journal of Issues in Nursing, 21*(1). http://ojin.nursingworld.org/MainMenuCategories/ANAMarketplace/ANAPeriodicals/OJIN/TableofContents/Vol-21-2016/No1-Jan-2016/The-Patient-Experience-and-Patient-Satisfaction.html

Gibson, K., Costa, B., & Sampson, A. (2017). *Linking worker health and safety with patient outcomes: A systematic review.* The Institute of Safety, Compensation and Recovery Research website: http://www.iscrr.com.au/__data/assets/pdf_file/0006/1321719/Evidence-Review_Linking-worker-health-and-safety-with-patient-outcomes.pdf

Jones, V., Missar, V., Bronson, M., & Grant, J. (2016). *Aon health care workers compensation barometer.* Aon.

Jones, V., Missar, V., Zmyslowski, K., Cregg, H., & Zhang, K. (2018). *Aon health care workers compensation barometer* (GDM08049). Aon.

Loeppke, R., Boldrighini, J., Bowe, J., Braun, B., Eggins, E., Eisenberg, B. S., Grundy, P., Hohn, T., Hudson, T. W., Kannas Jr., J., Kapp, E. A., Konicki, D., Larson, P., McCutcheon, S., McLellan, R. K., Ording, J., Perkins, C., Russi, M., Stutts, C., &

Yarbrough, M. (2017). Interaction of health care worker health and safety and patient health and safety in the US health care system: Recommendations from the 2016 Summit. *Journal of Occupational and Environmental Medicine, 59,* 803–813. https://doi.org/10.1097/JOM.0000000000001100

Matz, M., Celona, J., Martin, M., McCoskey, K., & Nelson, G. G. (2019). *Patient handling and mobility assessments.* (2nd ed.). The Facilities Guidelines Institute website: https://www.fgiguidelines.org/wp-content/uploads/2019/10/FGI-Patient-Handling-and-Mobility-Assessments_191008.pdf

Occupational Safety and Health Administration. (2013). *Safe patient handling programs: effectiveness and cost savings* (OSHA 3729 - 09/2013). https://www.osha.gov/Publications/OSHA3279.pdf

Teeple, E., Collins, J. E., Shrestha, S., Dennerlein, J. T., Losina, E., & Katz, J. N. (2017). Outcomes of safe patient handling and mobilization programs: A meta-analysis. *Work, 58,* 173–184. http://doi.org/10.3233/WOR-172608

7. POLICY/LEGISLATION

The ANA SPHM Interprofessional National Standards have continued to fill a void from the lack of federal safe patient handling and mobility (SPHM) regulations and in states without SPHM regulations. In 2015, a congressional SPHM bill was introduced by Representative John Conyers, Jr., known as the Nurse and Health Care Worker Protection Act of 2015. The bill died in committee. Two other attempts at legislation also died in committee.

Following a 3-year National Emphasis Program of planned inspections (2013–2015), which continued to highlight the high number of musculoskeletal injuries previously identified among healthcare workers in long-term care and residential facilities, OSHA issued a directive in 2015 for inpatient healthcare settings outlining specific SPHM program elements and policies to be reviewed when a facility received an OSHA compliance visit. The directive emphasized that healthcare consumer handling injuries were a recognized hazard as defined by OSHA and subject to regulatory oversight. General Duty clause violations and Hazard Alert letters continue to be written under this directive.

At the state level, no additional states have added SPHM legislation or resolutions since 2011. At present, 12 states have some form of legislation or resolution, of which nine require a comprehensive program. The states are California, Hawaii, Illinois, Maryland, Minnesota, Missouri, New Jersey, New York, Ohio, Rhode Island, Texas, and Washington (NIOSH, 2013).

Other standard promulgating bodies have also issued standards and guidelines related to SPHM programs. These include International Organization for Standardization (ISO) standard 10535:2021 Assistive products - Hoists for the transfer of disabled persons—Requirements and test methods and ISO/TR 12296:2012 Ergonomics—manual handling of people in the healthcare sector.

Guidelines for effective safety and management programs include ISO 45001 Occupational Health and Safety Management Systems 2018 and ANSI/ASSP Z10 Occupational Health and Safety Management Systems 2017. Elements in these standards may be applied when establishing any safety and health program, including SPHM.

REFERENCE

Centers for Disease Control and Prevention, National Institute for Occupational Safety and Health. (2013, August 2). *Safe patient handling and mobility (SPHM)*. https://www.cdc.gov/niosh/topics/safepatient/default.html

Organization and Intent of the Safe Patient Handling and Mobility Interprofessional National Standards

This is the second edition of the Safe Patient Handling and Mobility (SPHM) Interprofessional National Standards. The document contains eight overarching SPHM standards, each of which is organized into three parts: 1) standards addressing the responsibilities of the employer or healthcare organization, 2) standards addressing the responsibilities of the healthcare worker and ancillary/support staff, and 3) updated references related to the standard. Special considerations for community settings are also included to address current differences.

This document is designed to be used by many different professionals across the care continuum and is intended to be used across all healthcare settings and adapted by the user to specific settings, whenever possible.

The Advisory Group and Workgroup envisions that healthcare organizations may adopt these standards to improve the quality and safety of care, and to decrease and prevent injuries among healthcare workers and healthcare consumers. Insurance companies and other third-party payers may adopt these SPHM standards as an indication of quality and a condition of payment. Regulatory agencies may adopt or adapt these standards to control or improve the services of an industry. The SPHM standards may be used by the legal profession as evidence of the standard of care and to inform regulatory decisions.

The American Nurses Association and stakeholder contributors recognize that change takes time and resources, and recommend that organizations perform a SPHM needs assessment; establish priorities, goals, and objectives; develop a timeline for implementation and evaluation; and use the SPHM standards and references to create a safe environment of care.

NOTE: *The SPHM Interprofessional National Standards are open, voluntary standards. The standards do not require use of any specific products or services. ANA does not promote, endorse, or recommend any products or services.*

Safe Patient Handling and Mobility Interprofessional National Standards

STANDARD 1. ESTABLISH A CULTURE OF SAFETY

The employer and healthcare workers partner to establish a culture of safety that encompasses the core values and behaviors resulting from a collective and sustained commitment by organizational leadership, managers, healthcare workers, and ancillary/support staff to emphasize safety over competing goals.

1.1 EMPLOYER STANDARDS

Standard Number 1.1.1 Establish a Statement of Commitment to a Culture of Safety

Organizational policy will include a written commitment to a culture of safety that will be used to guide the organization's priorities, resource allocation, policies, and procedures. The written statement regarding safe patient handling and mobility (SPHM) will describe layers of accountability across sectors and settings.

Standard Number 1.1.2 Establish a Nonpunitive Environment

Organizational policy will support a system to encourage healthcare workers to report hazards, errors, incidents, and accidents, so that the precursors to SPHM errors can be better understood, and organizational issues can be changed to prevent future incidents and injuries. Healthcare workers know that they are accountable for their actions but will not be held accountable for problems within the system or environment that are beyond their control.

Standard Number 1.1.3 Provide a System for Right of Refusal

Organizational policy will provide the healthcare worker the right to accept, reject, or object to any healthcare consumer transfer, repositioning, or mobility assignment that puts the healthcare consumer or the healthcare worker at risk for injury. The refusal shall be made in writing, without fear of retribution. The policy will describe steps for resolving the hazard.

Standard Number 1.1.4 Provide Safe Levels of Staffing

An evidence-based system will be used to determine safe and appropriate caseloads. Adequate staffing levels will support safe patient handling and mobility, including allocated time for training and education.

Standard Number 1.1.5 Establish a System for Communication and Collaboration

Collaboration among all sectors and settings is critical. The organization will utilize a variety of effective communication systems to inform and engage the healthcare workers and healthcare consumers about SPHM.

1.2 HEALTHCARE WORKER STANDARDS

Standard Number 1.2.1 Participate in Creating and Maintaining a Culture of Safety

The healthcare worker will actively participate in creating and maintaining a culture of safety.

Standard Number 1.2.2 Notify the Employer of Hazards, Incidents, Near Misses, and Accidents

The healthcare worker will notify the employer of hazards, near misses, incidents, and accidents related to SPHM as soon as possible, using the reporting procedures defined by the employer.

Standard Number 1.2.3 Use The System to Communicate and Collaborate

The healthcare worker will engage, verbally, and in writing, with others about SPHM.

CONSIDERATIONS FOR COMMUNITY SETTINGS

The community setting provides unique challenges for the correction of hazards. For example, in home health, the healthcare worker is a guest in the home, and the healthcare consumer is typically financially responsible for the environment of care. Hazardous conditions, broken or inappropriate technology, or unreasonable requests must be discussed with the healthcare consumer and reported to the employer. The employer is ultimately responsible for the health of employees and can determine if engineering or other controls are available to correct the hazards or determine that care cannot be safely provided.

REFERENCES

American Nurses Association. (2009, March 12). *Patient safety: Rights of registered nurses when considering a patient assignment.* https://www.nursingworld.org/ practice-policy/nursing-excellence/official-position-statements/id/patient-safety-rights-of-registered-nurses-when-considering-a-patient-assignment/

American Nurses Association. (2010, January 28). *Just culture: ANA position statement.* https://www.nursingworld.org/practice-policy/nursing-excellence/ official-position-statements/id/just-culture/

American Nurses Association. (2016, May 4). American Nurses Association calls for a culture of safety in all health care settings. https://www.nursingworld.org/

news/news-releases/2016/american-nurses-association-calls-for-a-culture-of-safety-in-all-health-care-settings/

American Nurses Association. (2019). *Principles for nurse staffing*, (3rd ed). Author.

Elnitsky, C. A., Powell-Cope, G., Besterman-Dahan, K. L., Rugs, D., & Ullrich, P. M. (2015). Implementation of safe patient handling in the U.S. Veterans health system: A qualitative study of internal facilitators' perceptions. *Worldviews on Evidence-Based Nursing, 12,* 208–216. https://doi.org/10.1111/wvn.12098

Falco, K., & Monaghan, H. M. (2018). Soft skills: The foundation for effective SPHM program leadership: A national survey. *International Journal of Safe Patient Handling & Mobility, 8,* 76–99.

Gusenius, T. M., Decker, M. M., & Weidemann, A. G. (2018). Using shared governance to achieve a culture change in safe patient handling. *International Journal of Orthopaedic and Trauma Nursing, 31,* 35–39. https://doi.org/10.1016/j.ijotn.2018.07.002

Humrickhouse, R., & Knibbe, H. J. J. (2016). The importance of safe patient handling to create a culture of safety: An evidential review. *The Ergonomics Open Journal, 9,* 27–42. https://doi.org/10.2174/1875934301609010027

Institute for Healthcare Improvement. (n.d.). *Develop a culture of safety.* http://www.ihi.org/resources/Pages/Changes/DevelopaCultureofSafety.aspx

Koppelaar, E., Knibbe, J. J., Miedema, H. S., & Burdorf, A. (2013). The influence of individual and organisational factors on nurses' behaviour to use lifting devices in healthcare. *Applied Ergonomics, 44,* 532–537. https://doi.org/10.1016/j.apergo.2012.11.005

Morath, J. (2011). Nurses create a culture of patient safety: It takes more than projects. *Online Journal of Issues in Nursing, 16*(3), 2. https://doi.org/10.3912/OJIN.Vol16No03Man02

Stevens, L., Rees, S., Lamb, K. V., & Dalsing, D. (2013). Creating a culture of safety for safe patient handling. *Orthopaedic Nursing, 32,* 155–64. https://doi.org/10.1097/NOR.0b013e318291dbc5

STANDARD 2. IMPLEMENT AND SUSTAIN A SAFE PATIENT HANDLING AND MOBILITY PROGRAM

The employer and healthcare workers partner to establish a formal, systematized safe patient handling and mobility (SPHM) program for reducing the risk of injury to healthcare consumers and the risk of injuries and MSDs in healthcare workers, while improving the quality of care.

2.1 EMPLOYER STANDARDS

Standard Number 2.1.1 Designate a Group or Groups of Stakeholders to Develop, Implement, Evaluate, Remediate, and Maintain an SPHM Program

An organizational committee will identify or develop systems that support SPHM programs. The committee will receive and review data about SPHM and make recommendations for improvement. The work of the committee will reflect collaboration among organizational leadership, the healthcare workers who provide care for healthcare consumers, and ancillary/support workers.

Standard Number 2.1.2 Perform a Comprehensive Assessment of SPHM

The organization will initially and periodically perform a comprehensive assessment of patient handling, mobility, and technology, and SPHM program elements. Assessment will include an SPHM technology needs assessment (see Standard 4.1.1).

Standard Number 2.1.3 Develop a Written SPHM Program, With Goals, Objectives, and a Plan for Ongoing Evaluation, Compliance, and Quality Improvement

The written SPHM program will address each of the eight standards of Safe Patient Handling and Mobility: Interprofessional National Standards, and will reflect compliance with federal, state, and local laws and regulations. The written program will include short- and long-term goals and objectives, and a realistic plan and timeline to meet the goals and evaluation requirements. The written SPHM program will identify, by title, those individuals who have responsibility, authority, and accountability for developing and implementing the plan. The written SPHM program also will establish a clear reporting hierarchy to monitor compliance.

Standard Number 2.1.4 Customize and Integrate the SPHM Program Across the Continuum of Care

The SPHM program will be customized for, and integrated into, care settings throughout the organization and continuum of care, ensuring that SPHM is addressed through transitions of care. The organization will assist by identifying sources and funding strategies for varying types of SPHM technology that may be needed at transition from acute or long-term care.

Standard Number 2.1.5 Provide Funding to Implement and Sustain the Program

The employer will identify and allocate funding to implement and sustain the program based on business case and return-on-investment analytics or cost/benefit analysis.

Standard Number 2.1.6 Identify the Essential Physical Functions and High-Risk Tasks of Jobs

The organization will identify the essential physical functions of a job in a written job description. An evidence-based process or review of scientific literature will be used to identify activities that place the healthcare worker at high risk for injury, together with ergonomics evaluations of the performance of healthcare consumer care tasks.

Standard Number 2.1.7 Reduce the Physical Requirements of High-Risk Tasks

The organization will focus on reducing the physical requirements of high-risk transfer, repositioning, mobilization, and other applicable healthcare consumer tasks through ergonomic controls such as use of SPHM technology, safe work practices, and/or administrative controls.

2.2 HEALTHCARE WORKER STANDARDS

Standard Number 2.2.1 Participate in the SPHM Program

The healthcare worker will actively engage in the SPHM program, following the policies and procedures of the organization's SPHM program.

CONSIDERATIONS FOR COMMUNITY SETTINGS

The coordination of care at transition from acute or long-term care settings must address mobility needs. The healthcare consumer is often financially responsible for procurement of SPHM technology in home, community, and school settings; however, other methods of obtaining SPHM technology are available, e.g., provider prescription through Durable Medical Equipment (DME) through Medicare Part B, Veterans Health Administration (VHA), and/or community resources.

REFERENCES

Aslam, I., Davis, S. A., Feldman, S. R., & Martin, W. E. (2015). A review of patient lifting interventions to reduce health care worker injuries. *Workplace Health & Safety, 63*, 267–275. https://doi.org/10.1177/2165079915580038

Fragala, G., Boynton, T., Conti, M. T., Cyr, L., Enos, L., Kelly, D., McGann, N., Mullen, K., Salsbury, S., & Vollman, K. (2016, May 18). Patient-handling injuries: Risk factors and risk-reduction strategies. *American Nurse Today, 1*, 40–44. https://www.myamericannurse.com/patient-handling-injuries-risk-factors-risk-reduction-strategies/

Harwood, K., Darragh, A. R., Campo, M., Rockefeller, K., & Scalzetti, D. A. (2018). A systematic review of safe patient handling and mobility programs to prevent musculoskeletal injuries in occupational and physical therapists and assistants. *International Journal of Safe Patient Handling & Mobility, 8,* 46–55.

Hilton, T. (n.d.). *SPHM solutions everywhere for everyone: In the best interest of the patient and their caregivers.* U.S. Department of Veterans Affairs Public Health website: https://www.publichealth.va.gov/docs/employeehealth/SPHM-Solutions-Everywhere-for-Everyone.pdf#

International Organization for Standardization. (2012). *Ergonomics—Manual handling of people in the healthcare sector.* (ISO/TR 12296:2012). HTTPS://WWW.ISO.ORG/STANDARD/51310.HTML

Kanaskie, M. L., & Snyder, C. (2018). Nurses and nursing assistants decision-making regarding use of safe patient handling and mobility technology: A qualitative study. *Applied Nursing Research, 39,* 141–147. https://doi.org/10.1016/j.apnr.2017.11.006

Kucera, K. L., Schoenfisch, A. L., McIlvaine, J., Becherer, L., James, T., Yeung, Y. L., Avent, S., & Lipscomb, H. J. (2019). Factors associated with lift equipment use during patient lifts and transfers by hospital nurses and nursing care assistants: A prospective observational cohort study. *International Journal of Nursing Studies, 91,* 35–46. https://doi.org/10.1016/j.ijnurstu.2018.11.006

Kurowski, A., Buchholz, B., ProCare Research Team, & Punnett, L. (2014). A physical workload index to evaluate a safe resident handling program for nursing home personnel. *Human Factors, 56,* 669–683. https://doi.org/10.1177/0018720813509268

Kurowski, A., Gore, R., Roberts, Y., Kincaid, K. R., & Punnett, L. (2017). Injury rates before and after the implementation of a safe resident handling program in the long-term care sector. *Safety Science, 92,* 217–224. https://doi.org/10.1016/j.ssci.2016.10.012

Matz, M., Celona, J., Martin, M., McCoskey, K., & Nelson, G. G. (2019). *Patient handling and mobility assessments.* (2nd ed.). The Facility Guidelines Institute website: https://www.fgiguidelines.org/wp-content/uploads/2019/10/FGI-Patient-Handling-and-Mobility-Assessments_191008.pdf

Mayeda-Letourneau, J. (2014). Safe patient handling and movement: A literature review. *Rehabilitation Nursing, 39,* 123–129. https://doi.org/10.1002/rnj.133

Nelson, A., Matz, M., Chen, F., Siddharthan, K., Lloyd, J., & Fragala, G. (2006). Development and evaluation of a multifaceted ergonomics program to prevent injuries associated with patient handling tasks. *International Journal of Nursing Studies, 43,* 717–733. https://doi.org/10.1016/j.ijnurstu.2005.09.004

Parchem, K., Peck, A., & Tales, K. (2018). A multidisciplinary approach to equipment use in pediatric patient mobilization. *Critical Care Nursing Quarterly, 41,* 330–339. https://doi.org/10.1097/CNQ.0000000000000211

Park, S., Lavender, S. A., Sommerich, C. M., & Patterson, E. S. (2018). Increasing the use of patient lifting devices in nursing homes: Identifying the barriers and facilitators affecting the different adoption stages for an ergonomics intervention. *International Journal of Safe Patient Handling & Mobility, 8,* 9–24.

Powell-Cope, G., Toyinbo, P., Patel, N., Rugs, D., Elnitsky, C., Hahm, B., Sutton, B., Campbell, R., Besterman-Dahan, K., Matz, M., & Hodgson, M. (2014). Effects of a national safe patient handling program on nursing injury incidence rates. *Journal of Nursing Administration, 44, 525–534.* https://doi.org/10.1097/NNA.0000000000000111

Richardson, A., McNoe, B., Derrett, S., & Harcombe, H. (2018). Interventions to prevent and reduce the impact of musculoskeletal injuries among nurses: A systematic review. *International Journal of Nursing Studies, 82,* 58–67. https://doi.org/10.1016/j.ijnurstu.2018.03.018

Teeple, E., Collins, J. E., Shrestha, S., Dennerlein, J. T., Losina, E., & Katz, J. N. (2017). Outcomes of safe patient handling and mobilization programs: A meta-analysis. *Work, 58,* 173–184. https://doi.org/10.3233/WOR-172608

Thomas, D. R., & Thomas, Y. L. (2014). Interventions to reduce injuries when transferring patients: A critical appraisal of reviews and a realist synthesis. *International Journal of Nursing Studies, 51,* 1381–94. https://doi.org/10.1016/j.ijnurstu.2014.03.007

Totzkay, D. L. (2018). Multifactorial strategies for sustaining safe patient handling and mobility. *Critical Care Nursing Quarterly, 41,* 340–344. https://doi.org/10.1097/CNQ.0000000000000213

Veterans Health Administration Center for Engineering & Occupational Safety and Health. (2016). *Safe patient handling and mobility guidebook.* http://www.tampavaref.org/safe-patient-handling/implementation-tools.htm

Walker, L., Docherty, T., Hougendobler, D., Guanowsky, C., & Rosenthal, M. (2017). Sharing the lessons: The 10-year journey of a safe patient movement program. *International Journal of Safe Patient Handling & Mobility, 7,* 20–28.

STANDARD 3. INCORPORATE ERGONOMIC DESIGN PRINCIPLES TO PROVIDE A SAFE ENVIRONMENT OF CARE

The employer and healthcare workers partner to incorporate ergonomic design principles, such as those found in the design and construction of healthcare facilities' documents developed by the Facility Guidelines Institute, importantly, found within the *Patient Handling and Mobility Assessments*, 2nd Edition. Ergonomic design principles use a systematized and proactive process to prevent or reduce occupationally related illnesses, fatalities, and exposures by including prevention considerations in all designs that affect individuals in the occupational environment.

3.1 EMPLOYER STANDARDS
Standard Number 3.1.1 Plan for a Safe Environment of Care During New Construction And/Or Renovation
New construction and remodeling plans will incorporate a review of ergonomic and other safety and health risk factors into the design of all projects. These plans include considerations of facility design and process flow, evaluations of a variety of safe patient handling and mobility (SPHM) technology, and accessibility considerations.

Standard Number 3.1.2 Include Diverse Perspectives Related to Ergonomic Design Principles
Input will be gathered from healthcare workers and ancillary/support staff at all stages throughout all new construction, rebuilding, and remodeling activities.

3.2 HEALTHCARE WORKER STANDARDS
Standard Number 3.2.1 Provide Input into the Design
The healthcare worker and ancillary/support staff will provide input into the design of construction and remodeling projects.

CONSIDERATIONS FOR COMMUNITY SETTINGS
Ergonomic design principles must be applied in any healthcare setting undergoing construction or renovation.

REFERENCES
Devine, D. A., Wenger, B., Krugman, M., Zwink, J. E., Shiskowsky, K., Hagman, J., Limon, S., Snaders, C., & Reeves, C. (2015). Part 1: Evidence-based facility design using Transforming Care at the Bedside principles. *The Journal of Nursing Administration, 45*, 74–83. https://doi.org/10.1097/NNA.0000000000000161

Facility Guidelines Institute. (2018). Specific requirements for general hospitals: Bariatric patient care unit and Specific requirements for children's hospitals: Pediatric bariatric patient care unit. In *Guidelines for design and construction of hospitals*. Author.

Gallagher, S. M. (2013). *Implementation guide to the safe patient handling and mobility interprofessional national standards*. American Nurses Association.

Grant, M. P., Okechukwu, C. A., Hopcia, K., Sorensen, G., and Dennerlein, J. T. (2018). An inspection tool and process to identify modifiable aspects of acute care hospital patient care units to prevent work-related musculoskeletal disorders. *Workplace Health & Safety, 66,* 144–158. https://doi.org/10.1177/2165079917718852

Matz, M., Celona, J., Martin, M., McCoskey, K., & Nelson, G. G. (2019). *Patient handling and mobility assessments.* (2nd ed.). The Facilities Guidelines Institute website: https://www.fgiguidelines.org/wp-content/uploads/2019/10/FGI-Patient-Handling-and-Mobility-Assessments_191008.pdf

National Institute for Occupational Safety and Health. (2013). *Prevention through design (PtD)*. https://www.cdc.gov/niosh/topics/ptd/

STANDARD 4. SELECT, INSTALL, AND MAINTAIN SAFE PATIENT HANDLING AND MOBILITY TECHNOLOGY

The employer and healthcare workers partner to incorporate appropriate safe patient handling and mobility (SPHM) technology for the program. Such a program provides the assistive tools within the organization and at point-of-care that are used to facilitate SPHM, thus, minimizing the risk of injury to both the healthcare consumer and the healthcare worker. SPHM technology may include technology, devices, accessories, software, and multimedia resources.

4.1 EMPLOYER STANDARDS

Standard Number 4.1.1 Perform an Organizational SPHM Technology Needs Assessment

An interprofessional group of stakeholders and/or subject-matter experts will perform the organization's SPHM technology needs assessment within all environments of care.

Standard Number 4.1.2 Develop a Plan for the Selection of SPHM Technology

A plan will be identified to ensure that SPHM technology meets quality and safety standards, and that devices and accessories are compatible and interoperable within the organization or facility.

Standard Number 4.1.3 Provide Opportunities for Trial of and Provide Feedback on SPHM Technology

The organization considering the purchase or rental of SPHM technology will provide healthcare workers with opportunities to try out the technology and provide feedback.

Standard Number 4.1.4 Develop an SPHM Technology Procurement Plan and Introduction Schedule

The SPHM technology procurement plan and introduction schedule will be developed and communicated to the healthcare worker.

Standard Number 4.1.5 Provide and Strategically Place SPHM Technology for Accessibility

The organization will develop a process for providing SPHM technology that ensures ease in accessibility. The quantity and type of SPHM technology will be sufficient to minimize risk for the healthcare consumer population served and the environment of care.

Standard 4.1.6 Install Fixed SPHM Technology According to Manufacturer's Specifications

Fixed SPHM technology, such as ceiling- or wall-mounted lifts, or bariatric toilets will be installed according to the manufacturer's specifications.

Standard Number 4.1.7 Establish a System to Clean, Disinfect, Maintain, Repair, and Upgrade SPHM Technology

The employer will develop procedures for regular cleaning, disinfection, and maintenance. SPHM technology will be maintained and repaired according to the manufacturer's specifications. The responsibility for monitoring, and acting on, upgrade or recall notices for equipment or software will be assigned to a specific position.

4.2 HEALTHCARE WORKER STANDARDS

Standard Number 4.2.1 Participate in the SPHM Technology Needs Assessment

The healthcare worker will participate in the SPHM technology needs assessment and other processes, as appropriate.

Standard Number 4.2.2 Participate in SPHM Technology Selection

The healthcare worker will participate in the selection of technology as appropriate.

CONSIDERATIONS FOR COMMUNITY SETTINGS

A subject-matter expert in SPHM technology can provide solutions for specific problems or develop solutions for an entire organization. The SPHM technology industry continues to develop new technologies, work practices, and systems to meet the needs of users across the continuum of care. Newer technologies solve age-old problems like narrow doorways, small bathrooms, low beds, and steps. Healthcare consumers and their families must be encouraged to provide input regarding the usability, usefulness, and desirability of the SPHM technology options available to them.

REFERENCES

Association of periOperative Registered Nurses. (2021). Guideline for safe patient handling and movement. In: *Guidelines for Perioperative Practice.* Author.

Center for Health Design. (2014, 2017). *Safety risk assessment toolkit: A process to mitigate risk.* The Center for Health Design website: https://www.healthdesign.org/sra

Centers for Disease Control and Prevention. (2019). *Guidelines for environmental infection control in health-care facilities.* https://www.cdc.gov/infectioncontrol/pdf/guidelines/environmental-guidelines-P.pdf.

Dutta, T., Holliday, P. J., Gorski, S. M., Baharvandy, M. S., & Fernie, G. R. (2012). A biomechanical assessment of floor and overhead lifts using one or two caregivers for patient transfers. *Applied Ergonomics, 43,* 521–531. https://doi.org/10.1016/j.apergo.2011.08.006

Enos, L. (2018). The role of ceiling lifts in a safe patient handling and mobility program. *International Journal of Safe Patient Handling & Mobility, 8,* 25–45.

Enos, L. (2019). A comprehensive review of patient slings. *International Journal of Safe Patient Handling & Mobility, 9,* 15–36.

Gallagher, S., Alexandrowiz, M., Fritz, R., Kumpar, D., Miller, M., McNaughton, C., & Nowicki, T. (2020). Bariatric space, technology, and design: A round table. *Workplace Health & Safety, 68,* 313–319. https://doi.org/10.1177/2165079920911549

International Organization for Standardization. (2006). *Hoists for the transfer of disabled persons—Requirements and test methods.* (ISO 10535:2006). http://www.iso.org/standard/32155.html

International Organization for Standardization. (2012). *Ergonomics—Manual handling of people in the healthcare sector.* (ISO/TR 12296:2012). http://www.iso.org/iso/catalogue_detail.htm?csnumber=51310

Matz, M., Celona, J., Martin, M., McCoskey, K., & Nelson, G. G. (2019). *Patient handling and mobility assessments.* (2nd ed.).Facility Guidelines Institute website: https://www.fgiguidelines.org/wp-content/uploads/2019/10/FGI-Patient-Handling-and-Mobility-Assessments_191008.pdf

Monaghan, H. M. (2018). The role of mobile floor-based lifts in a safe patient handling and mobility program. *International Journal of Safe Patient Handling & Mobility, 8,* 91–99.

National Association of Orthopedic Nurses. *NEW! Safe patient handling algorithms.* http://www.orthonurse.org/p/bl/et/blogaid=926

Noble, N. L., & Sweeney, N. L. (2018). Barriers to the use of assistive devices in patient handling. *Workplace Health & Safety, 66,* 41–48. https://doi.org/10.1177/2165079917697216

Sedlak, C. A., Doheny, M. O., Nelson, A., & Waters, T. R. (2009). Development of the National Association of Orthopaedic Nurses guidance statement on safe patient handling and movement in the orthopaedic setting. *Orthopaedic Nursing, 28*(2S), S2–S8. https://doi.org/10.1097/NOR.0b013e318199c395

U.S. Department of Labor, Occupational Health and Safety Administration. (n.d.). Facility and patient needs assessment: Worker Safety in Hospitals. Worker Safety in Hospitals - Facility and Patient Needs Assessment | Occupational Safety and Health Administration (osha.gov)

U.S. Food & Drug Administration. (2018, August 22). *Medical Devices General Hospital—Devices and Supplies: Patient Lifts.* http://www.fda.gov/MedicalDevices/ProductsandMedicalProcedures/GeneralHospitalDevicesandSupplies/ucm308622.htm

U.S. Food & Drug Administration (FDA). (n.d.) (2021, August 12). Recalls, Market Withdrawals, & Safety [Data]. https://www.fda.gov/safety/recalls-market-withdrawals-safety-alerts

VHA Center for Engineering & Occupational Safety and Health. (2015). *Bariatric safe patient handling and mobility guidebook: A resource guide for care of persons of size.* http://www.tampavaref.org/safe-patient-handling/implementation-tools.htm

VHA Center for Engineering & Occupational Safety and Health. (2016). *Safe patient handling and mobility guidebook.* http://www.tampavaref.org/safe-patient-handling/implementation-tools.htm

Waters, T. R., Dick, R., Lowe, B., Werren, D., & Parsons, K. (2012). Ergonomic assessment of floor-based and overhead lifts. *American Journal of Safe Patient Handling & Movement, 2,* 119–133.

STANDARD 5. ESTABLISH A SYSTEM FOR EDUCATION, TRAINING, AND MAINTAINING COMPETENCE

The employer and healthcare workers partner to establish an effective system of education and training to maintain safe patient handling and mobility (SPHM) competence of healthcare workers and ancillary/support staff.

5.1 EMPLOYER STANDARDS

Standard Number 5.1.1 Establish an Education and Training System

SPHM education and training will be provided to the healthcare worker and ancillary/support staff as appropriate, at orientation, annually, and with the introduction of new competencies or technology solutions. Select a methodology that meets the needs of the adult learner.

Standard Number 5.1.2 Include Healthcare Workers from Across the Continuum of Care

The content of the education and training will be specific to the role and setting of the healthcare worker or ancillary/support staff.

Standard Number 5.1.3 Provide Time for Employees to Participate in Learning Sessions

Employee participation will be facilitated by providing time and scheduling support services. Education and training will be provided during scheduled work hours, including alternate shift work.

Standard Number 5.1.4 Provide Appropriate SPHM Technology for Education and Training

Interactive education and training will be conducted using the same types of SPHM technology used for healthcare consumer care within the organization. Simulation or point-of-care training is preferred.

Standard Number 5.1.5 Require and Document Healthcare Worker Competence

The healthcare worker will demonstrate competence with SPHM prior to providing actual care. The effectiveness of education and training will be monitored.

Standard Number 5.1.6 Provide Time and Resources for the Education of Healthcare Consumers

The organization will allocate time and learning resources for healthcare workers to educate healthcare consumers and their families about SPHM, as appropriate.

5.2 HEALTHCARE WORKER STANDARDS

Standard Number 5.2.1 Establish and Maintain Competence

The healthcare worker will actively participate in education and training to maintain competence related to SPHM and serve as a role model for safe behavior.

Standard Number 5.2.2 Engage and Educate the Healthcare Consumer Regarding SPHM

The healthcare worker will engage and educate healthcare consumers, family, community, and co-workers in a manner that is easily understood by the learner.

CONSIDERATIONS FOR COMMUNITY SETTINGS

Healthcare workers employed in community settings such as home health agencies, congregant care, or schools may encounter a wide variety of SPHM technology. When new SPHM technology will be used, training should be provided at the point of care, and the employer must ensure that the healthcare worker has access to a subject-matter expert for questions or consultation. Periodic updates with SPHM technology vendors or a local durable medical goods vendor may be helpful and would provide a time for evaluative feedback on the special needs of community settings.

REFERENCES

Alamgir, H., Drebit, S., Li, H. G., Kidd, C., Tam, H., & Fast, C. (2011). Peer coaching and mentoring: A new model of educational intervention for safe patient handling in health care. *American Journal of Industrial Medicine, 54,* 609–617. https://doi.org/10.1002/ajim.20968

Boucaut, R., & Howson, D. (2018). Teaching safe patient handling skills using a peer approach. *Radiologic Technology, 90,* 20–30.

Fitzpatrick, M. A. (2014). Safe patient handling and mobility: A call to action. *American Nurse Journal.* https://www.myamericannurse.com/wp-content/uploads/2014/07/ant9-Patient-Handling-Supplement-821a_LOW.pdf

Gallagher, S. M. (2012). Intergenerational considerations in sustaining safe patient handling and mobility success: Implications in equipment usage. *International Journal of Safe Patient Handling & Mobility, 2,* 134–137.

Hogan, D. A. M., Greiner, B.A., & O'Sullivan, L. (2014). The effect of manual handling training on transferring knowledge, employee's behaviour change and subsequent reduction of work-related musculoskeletal disorders: A systematic review. *Ergonomics, 5,* 93–107. https://doi.org/10.1080/00140139.2013.862307

Jacobs, R., Beyer, E., & Carter, K. (2017). Interprofessional simulation education designed to teach occupational therapy and nursing students complex patient transfers. *Journal of Interprofessional Education & Practice, 6,* 67–70. https://doi.org/10.1016/j.xjep.2016.12.002

Lee, C., Knight, S. W., Smith, S. L., Nagle, D. J., & DeVries, L. (2018). Safe patient handling and mobility: Development and implementation of a large-scale education program. *Critical Care Nursing Quarterly, 41,* 253–263. https://doi.org/10.1097/CNQ.0000000000000204

Matz, M., Celona, J., Martin, M., McCoskey, K., & Nelson, G. G. (2019) *Patient Handling and Mobility Assessments*. (2nd ed.). Facilities Guidelines Institute website: https://www.fgiguidelines.org/wp-content/uploads/2019/10/FGI-Patient-Handling-and-Mobility-Assessments_191008.pdf

Monaghan, H. M. (2019). Making safe patient handling and mobility training effective. Part 1. What to teach, where and when to teach it and how to teach it. *International Journal of Safe Patient Handling & Mobility, 9*, 143–148.

Monaghan, H. M. (2020). Making safe patient handling and mobility training effective. Part 2. Assessing competent practice. *International Journal of Safe Patient Handling & Mobility, 10*, 37–41.

Noble, N. L., & Sweeney, N. L. (2018). Barriers to the use of assistive devices in patient handling. *Workplace Health & Safety, 66*, 41–48. https://doi.org/10.1177/2165079917697216

Perez, A. (2016). An evidence-based approach to safe patient handling and mobility education. *International Journal of Safe Patient Handling & Mobility, 6*, 113–119.

Powell-Cope, G., Pippins, K. M., & Young, H. M. (2017). Teaching family caregivers to assist safely with mobility. *American Journal of Nursing, 117*(12), 49–53. https://doi.org/10.1097/01.NAJ.0000527485.94115.7e

Roberts, T. (2020). Simulation to teach safe patient handling and mobility for home caregivers. *Home Health Care Management & Practice, 32*, 206–210. https://doi.org/10.1177/1084822320925801

Wanless, S. (2017). Applying theories of health behavior and change to moving and handling practice. *International Journal of Safe Patient Handling & Mobility, 7*, 105–109.

Wright, D. K. (2005). *The Ultimate Guide to Competency Assessment in Health Care* (3rd ed). Creative Health Care Management.

STANDARD 6. INTEGRATE PATIENT-CENTERED SAFE PATIENT HANDLING AND MOBILITY ASSESSMENT, PLAN OF CARE, AND USE OF SAFE PATIENT HANDLING AND MOBILITY TECHNOLOGY

The employer and healthcare workers partner to adapt the plan of care to meet the safe patient handling and mobility (SPHM) needs of individual healthcare consumers and specify appropriate SPHM technology and methods.

6.1 EMPLOYER STANDARDS

Standard Number 6.1.1 Provide a Written Procedure on the SPHM Assessment and Plan of Care

The written procedure outlines how to evaluate a healthcare consumer's SPHM status, establish goals, select technology for specific care tasks, and address roles and responsibilities of the healthcare worker related to assessment and scoring, evaluation, plan of care, and documentation.

Standard Number 6.1.2 Require Initial and Ongoing Assessment or Process to Determine SPHM Needs

The healthcare consumer will be evaluated for physical, cognitive, clinical, and rehabilitative needs that impact mobility and other healthcare consumer handling and care needs, both initially and on an ongoing basis. The outcome of the assessment, evaluation, or scoring system will be incorporated within the individual plan of care.

Standard Number 6.1.3 Include SPHM in the Plan of Care

The individual plan of care will specify required SPHM technology and methods and expected outcomes. The plan of care should promote the healthcare consumer's independence or return to baseline as appropriate.

Standard Number 6.1.4 Address SPHM at Transitions of Care

The shift report, transfer, or discharge plan will include information and resources for SPHM, as appropriate.

Standard Number 6.1.5 Provide a System to Resolve Healthcare Consumer's Refusal

A system must be developed to address the safety of the healthcare worker and the healthcare consumer if the healthcare consumer refuses the use of SPHM technology.

Standard Number 6.1.6 Monitor Healthcare Consumer Injuries Associated with Patient Handling and Mobility

The organization will determine the type, frequency, severity, and cost of healthcare consumer injuries associated with patient handling and mobility.

Standard Number 6.1.7 Support Safe Delegation of SPHM Tasks and Activities

The organization will support the delegation or assignment in a manner consistent with its state's practice act or other legislation governing licensure.

6.2 HEALTHCARE WORKER STANDARDS

Standard Number 6.2.1 Perform Initial and Ongoing Assessment of Mobility and SPHM Needs

The healthcare worker will perform initial and ongoing assessments of mobility and SPHM needs, as per organizational policy.

Standard Number 6.2.2 Communicate With the Healthcare Consumer and Family

The healthcare worker will educate the healthcare consumer and family, as appropriate, about the purposes and safe use of SPHM technology.

Standard Number 6.2.3 Address SPHM at Transitions of Care

The healthcare worker will include SPHM in shift reports, transfer reports, and discharge planning.

Standard Number 6.2.4 Delegate Care Tasks in a Safe Manner

The healthcare worker will ensure that delegation or assignment of SPHM tasks is completed in a manner consistent with state professional practice acts or other applicable laws or regulations.

CONSIDERATIONS FOR COMMUNITY SETTINGS

The healthcare worker will provide information on appropriate and available SPHM technologies and supplies. Healthcare consumers and their families must be central to the process of selection. Helping the family understand the importance of the SPHM technology is critical in obtaining their "buy-in." The use of SPHM technology in long-term care, and specifically in assisted living settings, is an important part of promoting independence. Progression through different technologies may indicate a functional change: possibly deterioration, possibly improvement.

REFERENCES

American Nurses Association. (2021). *Nursing scope and standards of practice* (4th ed.). Author.

Arnold, M. (2019). Functional assessments for safe patient mobilization across the continuum of care. *International Journal of Safe Patient Handling & Mobility, 9,* 111–121.

Association of periOperative Registered Nurses. (2021). Guideline for safe patient handling and movement. In: *Guidelines for Perioperative Practice.* Author.

Boynton, T., Kumpar, D., & VanGilder, C. (2020). The bedside mobility assessment tool 2.0. *American Nurse Journal, 15*(7), 18–22. https://www.myamericannurse.com/wp-content/uploads/2020/06/an7-Mobility-618.pdf

Dickinson, S., Taylor, S., & Anton, P. (2018). Integrating a standardized mobility program and safe patient handling. *Critical Care Nursing Quarterly, 41,* 240–252. https://doi.org/ 10.1097/CNQ.0000000000000202

Gallagher, S. (2015). *A practical guide to bariatric safe patient handling & mobility: Improving safety and quality for the patient of size.* Visioning Publishers.

Gallagher, S., Hilton, T., Monaghan, H. M., Muir, M., & Dye, A. (2014). Safe patient handling and movement: Bariatric considerations. *International Journal of Safe Patient Handling & Movement, 4*(2), S1–S16.

Harwood, K. J., Scalzitti, D. A., Campo, M., & Darragh, A. R. (2016). A systematic review of safe patient handling and mobility programs to improve patient outcomes in rehabilitation. *International Journal of Safe Patient Handling & Movement, 6,* 141–150.

Matthews, J. H., & Bruflat, C. M. (2010). *ANA's principles for nursing documentation: Guidance for registered nurses.* American Nurses Association, Nursesbooks.

Matz, M., Celona, J., Martin, M., McCoskey, K., & Nelson, G. G. (2019). *Patient handling and mobility assessments.* (2nd ed.). The Facilities Guidelines Institute website: https://www.fgiguidelines.org/wp-content/uploads/2019/10/FGI-Patient-Handling-and-Mobility-Assessments_191008.pdf

Sedlak, C. A., Doheny, M. O., Nelson, A., & Waters, T. R. (2009). Development of the National Association of Orthopaedic Nurses guidance statement on safe patient handling and movement in the orthopaedic setting. *Orthopaedic Nursing, 28*(2S), S2–S8. https://doi.org/10.1097/NOR.0b013e318199c395

VHA Center for Engineering & Occupational Safety and Health. (2016). *Safe patient handling and mobility guidebook.* http://www.tampavaref.org/safe-patient-handling/implementation-tools.htm

Wang, S., Hammes, J., Khan, S., Gao, S., Harrawood, A., Martinez, S., Moser, L., Perkins, A., Unverzagt, F.W., Clark., D.O., Boustani, M., & Khan, B. (2018). Improving recovery and outcomes every day after the ICU (IMPROVE): Study protocol for a randomized controlled trial. *Trials, 19, 196.* https://doi.org/10.1186/s13063-018-2569-8

Yeung, Y. (2015). Increase access to healthcare services with safe patient handling and mobility equipment. *International Journal of Safe Patient Handling & Movement, 5,* 104–147.

STANDARD 7. INCLUDE SAFE PATIENT HANDLING AND MOBILITY IN REASONABLE ACCOMMODATION AND POST-OCCUPATIONAL INJURY RETURN TO WORK

The employer and healthcare workers partner to establish a comprehensive safe patient handling and mobility (SPHM) program that can help the employer provide reasonable accommodations to healthcare workers who are injured at work.

7.1 EMPLOYER STANDARDS

Standard Number 7.1.1 Facilitate the Safe Utilization of Injured Workers

The organization will have a system to match the physical capability of an injured healthcare worker to the physical demands of a job. The use of safe patient handling and mobility (SPHM) technology is one strategy to facilitate the safe utilization of injured workers.

Standard Number 7.1.2 Monitor Healthcare Worker Injuries Associated With Patient Handling and Mobility

Monitoring will include determining the frequency, severity, and cost of healthcare worker injuries associated with lifting, transfers, repositioning, mobility, and other high-risk care of healthcare consumers. Data about healthcare worker injuries will be used to prevent future injuries.

Standard Number 7.1.3 Facilitate Safe Early Return to Work Following Injury

The employer will establish, implement, and sustain a process to help injured healthcare workers return to work as quickly as possible to jobs that are medically suited to their needs. The process will be managed to ensure that restrictions are honored, preventing harm, and expediting recovery during the restricted work activity period.

7.2 HEALTHCARE WORKER STANDARDS

Standard Number 7.2.1 Notify the Employer of Physical Limitations or Restrictions

The healthcare worker will notify the employer of any physical limitations and provide up-to-date medical documentation of physical limitations or restrictions.

Standard Number 7.2.2 Participate in the Return-To-Work Plan

The injured healthcare worker will be accountable for complying with the medical treatment plan and for returning to work in a role that accommodates medical restrictions.

CONSIDERATIONS FOR COMMUNITY SETTINGS

Every healthcare organization will have a system for evaluating, managing, and reducing healthcare worker injuries.

REFERENCES

Baptiste, A. (2011). An evaluation of nursing tasks. *Work, 40,* 115–124. https://doi.org/10.3233/WOR-2011-1213

Cancelliere, C., Donovan, J., Stochkendahl, M. J., Biscardi, M., Ammendolia, C., Myburgh, C., & Cassidy, J. D. (2016). Factors affecting return to work after injury or illness: Best evidence synthesis of systematic reviews. *Chiropractic & Manual Therapies, 24,* 1–23. https://doi.org/10.1186/s12998-016-0113-z

Centers for Disease Control and Prevention, National Institute for Occupational Safety and Health. (2013, August 2). *Safe patient handling and mobility (SPHM).* https://www.cdc.gov/niosh/topics/safepatient/default.html

Centers for Disease Control and Prevention, National Institute for Occupational Safety and Health. (2018, November 2). *Elements of ergonomic programs. Step 6: Promote worker recovery through health care management and return-to-work.* https://www.cdc.gov/niosh/topics/ergonomics/ergoprimer/step6.html

Cullen, K. L., Irvin, E., Collie, A., Clay, F., Gensby, U., Jennings, P. A., Hogg-Johnson, S., Kristman, V., Laberge, M., McKenzie, D., Newman, S., Palagyi, A., Ruseckaite, R., Sheppard, D.M., Shourie, S., Steenstra, I., Van Eerd, D., & Amick, B. C. (2018). Effectiveness of workplace interventions in return-to-work for musculoskeletal, pain-related and mental health conditions: An update of the evidence and messages for practitioners. *Journal of Occupational Rehabilitation, 28,* 1–15. https://doi.org/10.1007/s10926-016-9690-x

Etuknwa, A., Daniels, K., & Eib, C. (2019). Sustainable return to work: A systematic review focusing on personal and social factors. *Journal of Occupational Rehabilitation, 29,* 679–700. https://doi.org/10.1007/s10926-019-09832-7

Grant, M., O'Beirne-Elliman, J., Froud, R., Underwood, M., & Seers, K. (2019). The work of return to work. Challenges of returning to work when you have chronic pain: A meta-ethnography. *BMJ Open, 9*(6), e025743. https://doi.org/10.1136/bmjopen-2018-025743

Kurowski, A., Pransky, G., & Punnett, L. (2019). Impact of a safe resident handling program in nursing homes on return-to-work and re-injury outcomes following work injury. *Journal of Occupational Rehabilitation, 29,* 286–294. https://doi.org/10.1007/s10926-018-9785-7

Matz, M., Celona, J., Martin, M., McCoskey, K., & Nelson, G. G. (2019). *Patient handling and mobility assessments.* (2nd ed.). The Facilities Guidelines Institute website: https://www.fgiguidelines.org/wp-content/uploads/2019/10/FGI-Patient-Handling-and-Mobility-Assessments_191008.pdf

National Association of Orthopedic Nurses. NEW! Safe Patient Handling Algorithms. NAON. http://www.orthonurse.org/p/bl/et/blogaid=926

Sedlak, C. A., Doheny, M. O., Nelson, A., & Waters, T. R. (2009). Development of the National Association of Orthopaedic Nurses guidance statement on safe patient handling and movement in the orthopaedic setting. *Orthopaedic Nursing, 28*(2S), S2–S8. https://doi.org/10.1097/NOR.0b013e318199c395

Shaw, W. S., Nelson, C. C., Woiszwillo, M. J., Gaines, B., & Peters, S. E. (2018). Early return to work has benefits for relief of back pain and functional recovery after controlling for multiple confounds. *Journal of Occupational and Environmental Medicine, 60*, 901–910. https://doi.org/10.1097/JOM.0000000000001380

United States. (1990). Americans with Disabilities Act of 1990. Public Law No. 101-336. *United States Statutes at Large*, 104, 327. https://www.govinfo.gov/content/pkg/STATUTE-104/pdf/STATUTE-104-Pg327.pdf

United States Department of Labor, Occupational Safety and Health Administration. *OSHA injury and illness recordkeeping and reporting requirements*. Retrieved August 13, 2020, from https://www.osha.gov/recordkeeping

Waters, T. R. (2007). When is it safe to manually lift a patient? *American Journal of Nursing, 107*(8), 53–58. https://doi.org/10.1097/01.NAJ.0000282296.18688.b1

STANDARD 8. ESTABLISH A COMPREHENSIVE EVALUATION SYSTEM

The employer and healthcare workers partner to establish a comprehensive system to evaluate safe patient handling and mobility (SPHM) program outcomes, trends, and processes, including staff performance, engagement, and compliance; staff injury incidence and severity; effectiveness of technology; and healthcare consumer outcome metrics.

8.1 EMPLOYER STANDARDS

Standard Number 8.1.1 Establish a Comprehensive Evaluation System

The organization will establish a comprehensive evaluation and performance/ quality improvement system during the planning phase of the SPHM program, based on the goals and objectives of the SPHM program. Formative and summative evaluations will be performed, including process and outcome measures. Evaluations will be conducted on a regular basis. The program evaluation methods will change depending on the maturity of the SPHM program. A mechanism will be used to provide organizational leadership and key stakeholders with the results of these analyses. Positive outcomes will be emphasized, and remediation plans will be developed for substandard outcomes.

Standard Number 8.1.2 Identify a Variety of Data Sources and Measures

The organization will identify appropriate organizational performance/quality improvement indicators that reflect the content of Safe Patient Handling and Mobility: Interprofessional National Standards, assess the effectiveness of the SPHM program and the processes implemented during program development, and identify selected program outcomes.

Standard Number 8.1.3 Utilize Evidence-Based Methods for Data Collection and Analysis

The organization will use standardized definitions and evidence-based methods for data collection and analysis. Evaluation methods may change depending on the maturity of the SPHM program.

Standard Number 8.1.4 Disseminate Findings

The organization establishes a formal process of informing all stakeholders of the SPHM outcomes using a variety of techniques, including, but not limited to, online summary of data; printed materials distributed to the healthcare worker; and regularly scheduled meetings, management meetings, and organizational meetings (see Standard 1.1.5).

Standard Number 8.1.5 Develop a Plan for Performance/Quality Improvement and Remediation of Deficiencies

A diverse group of stakeholders (Standard 2.1.1) will review the data and develop recommendations. The organization will develop and implement a plan or activities to remediate deficiencies within a reasonable time.

Standard Number 8.1.6 Comply With the Organization's Policies, Professional Codes of Ethics, Privacy Laws and Regulations, and Other Regulatory Language

The SPHM program will comply with organizational policies, appropriate professional codes of ethics, the Health Insurance Portability Privacy and Accountability Act, the Americans with Disabilities Act, state workers' compensation laws, and other applicable codes and regulations.

8.2 HEALTHCARE WORKER STANDARDS
Standard Number 8.2.1 Assist With Data Collection

The healthcare worker will provide accurate information during data collection and communication of results.

Standard Number 8.2.2 Comply With the Organization's Policies, Professional Codes of Ethics, Privacy Laws and Regulations, and Other Regulatory Language

The healthcare worker will be accountable for knowing and following the policies of the organization, following a professional code of ethics, and respecting the privacy of healthcare consumers and co-workers.

CONSIDERATIONS FOR COMMUNITY SETTINGS

Every healthcare organization will have a system for evaluating and improving the effectiveness of the SPHM program.

REFERENCES

American Industrial Hygiene Association. (2014). *AIHA/OSHA Alliance tip sheet—safe patient handling and mobility.* OSHA-Quick-Tips-on-SPHM_Final-Mar2014.pdf (digitaloceanspaces.com) and https://aiha-assets.sfo2.digitaloceanspaces.com/AIHA/resources/Quick-Tips-on-SPHM-Spanish-OSHA-review-6-27-14_FINAL.pdf

American Industrial Hygiene Association. (2019). *The facts about ergonomics: Dispelling myths: Position statement.* https://aiha-assets.sfo2.digitaloceanspaces.com/AIHA/resources/Position-Statements/Facts-About-Ergonomics-Dispelling-Myths-Position-Statement.pdf

American Industrial Hygiene Association. *AIHA Value Strategy* TVS Associates. http://www.tvsassociates.com/AIHA_Value_Strategy.html

Association of Safe Patient Handling Professionals. (2017). *Legislative update.* https://asphp.org/resources-tools/legislative-updates/

California A. B. 1136, Bill Text—AB-1136. Employment safety: Health facilities. http://leginfo.legislature.ca.gov/faces/billTextClient.xhtml?bill_id=201120120AB1136

International Organization for Standardization. (2018). *Occupational health and safety management system—Requirements with guidance for use.* (ISO 45001:2018). https://www.iso.org/standard/63787.html

Jones, R. (2017). ISO 45001 and the evolution of occupational health and safety management systems. *IOSH—Institution of Occupational Safety and Health Paper*, 1–7. ISO 45001 and the evolution of occupational health and safety management systems (iosh.com)

Matz, M., Celona, J., Martin, M., McCoskey, K., & Nelson, G. G. (2019). *Patient handling and mobility assessments.* (2nd ed.). The Facilities Guidelines Institute website: https://www.fgiguidelines.org/wp-content/uploads/2019/10/FGI-Patient-Handling-and-Mobility-Assessments_191008.pdf

Occupational Safety and Health Administration. (n.d.). *Safe patient handling: A self-assessment.* https://www.osha.gov/sites/default/files/3.8_SPH_self-assessment_508.pdf

U.S. Food and Drug Administration. (2014, September 8). *Corrective and preventive actions (CAPA).* https://www.fda.gov/corrective-and-preventive-actions-capa

VHA Center for Engineering & Occupational Safety and Health. (2016). *Safe patient handling and mobility guidebook.* http://www.tampavaref.org/safe-patient-handling/implementation-tools.htm

Resources — Safe Patient Handling and Mobility (SPHM)

INTRODUCTION

The materials listed here are suggested as sources for further information. Several of these documents were used to inform the development of the Safe Patient Handling and Mobility Interprofessional National Standards. This list is a highlight of available information and is not meant to represent a comprehensive list of available SPHM publications and programs. Many of these references are also cited throughout the document. Resources are listed by relevance to each Standard.

STANDARD 1. ESTABLISH A CULTURE OF SAFETY

- **American Nurses Association Calls for a Culture of Safety in All Health Care Settings** American Nurses Association (ANA), 2016. https://www.nursingworld.org/news/news-releases/2016/american-nurses-association-calls-for-a-culture-of-safety-in-all-health-care-settings/

- **Develop a Culture of Safety and Other Safety Improvement Tools.** *Website with Multiple Resources.* Institute for Healthcare Improvement (IHI). http://www.ihi.org/resources/Pages/Changes/DevelopaCultureofSafety.aspx

- **Development and Evaluation of a Multifaceted Ergonomics Program to Prevent Injuries Associated With Patient Handling Tasks.** Nelson, A. et al. International Journal of Nursing Studies, 43(6), 717–733. 2006. https://digitalcommons.unl.edu/cgi/viewcontent.cgi?referer=&httpsredir=1&article=1058&context=veterans

- **Every Injury to a Health Care Worker Is Preventable.** Gerwig, K. Institute of Healthcare Improvement (IHI). Wednesday, January 22, 2020. http://www.ihi.org/communities/blogs/every-injury-to-a-health-care-worker-is-preventable

- **Fundamentals of Total Worker Health® Approaches Essential Elements for Advancing Worker Safety, Health, and Well-Being.** National Institute for Occupational Safety and Health (NIOSH), 2016. https://www.cdc.gov/niosh/docs/2017-112/pdfs/2017_112.pdf

- **Handle With Care®.** *Website with Multiple Resources.* American Nurses Association (ANA). https://www.nursingworld.org/practice-policy/work-environment/health-safety/handle-with-care

- **Health Nurse Healthy Nation Year 3 Highlights 2019–2020.** American Journal of Nursing Sept. 2020 3–11. https://www.healthynursehealthynation.org/globalassets/all-images-view-with-media/about/2019-hnhn_highlights.pdf

- **Health Nurse Healthy Nation Highlights 2018–2019.** American Journal of Nursing Sept. 2019 3–11. https://www.healthynursehealthynation.org/globalassets/all-images-view-with-media/about/2020-hnhn_sup-8.pdf
- **IHI Framework for Improving Joy in Work.** Perlo J., Balik B., Swensen S., Kabcenell A., Landsman J., & Feeley D. IHI White Paper. Cambridge, Massachusetts: Institute for Healthcare Improvement (IHI), 2017. http://www.ihi.org/resources/Pages/IHIWhitePapers/Framework-Improving-Joy-in-Work.aspx
- **Implementation of Safe Patient Handling in the US Veterans Health System: A Qualitative Study of Internal Facilitators' Perceptions.** Elnitsky, C. A., Powell-Cope, G., Besterman-Dahan, K. L., Rugs, D., & Ullrich, P. M. *Worldviews on Evidence-Based Nursing, 12*(4), 208–216.2015. https://www.nursingcenter.com/ce_articleprint?an=00000446-201811000-00023
- **Improving Patient and Worker Safety: Opportunities for Synergy, Collaboration and Innovation.** The Joint Commission (TJC), 2012. https://www.jointcommission.org/-/media/tjc/documents/resources/patient-safety-topics/patient-safety/tjc-improvingpatientandworkersafety-monograph.pdf
- **Interaction of Health Care Worker Health and Safety and Patient Health and Safety in the US Health Care System: Recommendations From the 2016 Summit.** Loeppke, R. et al. American College of Occupational and Environmental Medicine (ACOEM) Position Statement. Journal of Occupational and Environmental Medicine, 59(8), 803–813. 2017. http://www.acoem.org/uploadedFiles/Public_Affairs/Policies_And_Position_Statements/Guidelines/Position_Statements/Interaction_of_Health_Care_Worker_Health_and.17.pdf
- **Just Culture Position Statement.** American Nurses Association (ANA), January 28, 2010. https://www.nursingworld.org/practice-policy/nursing-excellence/official-position-statements/id/just-culture/#:~:text=ANA%20supports%20the%20Just%20Culture%20concept%20and%20its,in%20developing%20regional%20and%20state-wide%20Just%20Culture%20initiatives
- **Just Culture: It's More Than Policy.** Paradiso, L., & Sweeney, N. Nursing Management (Springhouse): 50(6), 38–45. 2019. https://journals.lww.com/nursingmanagement/Fulltext/2019/06000/Just_culture__It_s_more_than_policy.9.aspx
- **Leading a Culture of Safety: A Blueprint for Success.** American College of Healthcare Executives (ACHE). Institute for Healthcare Improvement NPSF, 2017. https://www.osha.gov/shpguidelines/docs/Leading_a_Culture_of_Safety-A_Blueprint_for_Success.pdf
- **Linking Worker Health and Safety with Patient Outcomes.** Gibson, K., Costa, B., & Sampson, A. WorkSafe Victoria (WSV). The Institute of Safety, Compensation and Recovery Research (ISCRR). 2017. http://www.iscrr.

com.au/__data/assets/pdf_file/0006/1321719/Evidence-Review_Linking-worker-health-and-safety-with-patient-outcomes.pdf

- **Measuring Best Practices for Workplace Safety, Health, and Well-Being. The Workplace Integrated Safety and Health Assessment**. Sorensen, G., Sparer, E., Williams, J. A., Gundersen, D., Boden, L. I., Dennerlein, J. T., . . . & Pronk, N. P. Journal of Occupational and Environmental Medicine, 60(5), 430–439. 2018.https://www.ncbi.nlm.nih.gov/pmc/articles/PMC5943154/

- **Missed Nursing Care.** Agency for Healthcare Research and Quality (AHRQ). AHRQ PSNet Patient Safety Primer. Updated Sept. 2019, https://psnet.ahrq.gov/primer/missed-nursing-care

- **Nurses Create a Culture of Patient Safety: It Takes More Than Projects.** Morath, J. American Nurses Association (ANA), *OJIN*. September 3, 2015. http://ojin.nursingworld.org/MainMenuCategories/ANAMarketplace/ANAPeriodicals/OJIN/TableofContents/Vol-16-2011/No3-Sept-2011/Nurses-Create-a-Culture-of-Patient-Safety.aspx#:~:text=Nurses%20play%20an%20essential%20role%20in%20developing%20the,provide%20leadership%20to%20strengthen%20the%20culture%20of%20safety

- **Patient-Handling Injuries: Risk Factors and Risk-Reduction Strategies.** Fragala et al. American Nurse Today. 11(5):40–43. 2016. https://www.myamericannurse.com/wp-content/uploads/2016/05/Patient-Handling-Safety-426b.pdf

- **Patient Safety: Rights of Registered Nurses When Considering a Patient Assignment**. American Nurses Association (ANA). March 12, 2009. https://www.nursingworld.org/practice-policy/nursing-excellence/official-position-statements/id/patient-safety-rights-of-registered-nurses-when-considering-a-patient-assignment/#:~:text=The%20American%20Nurses%20Association%20%28ANA%29%20upholds%20that%20registered,patients%20or%20themselves%20at%20serious%20risk%20for%20harm

- **Principles of Safe Staffing**, ANA, 2019, 3rd ed. American Nurses Association (ANA), https://www.nursingworld.org/practice-policy/nurse-staffing/staffing-principles/

- **Recommended practices for Safety and Health Programs.** OSHA 3885. Occupational Safety and Health Administration (OSHA), 2016. https://www.osha.gov/Publications/OSHA3885.pdf

- **Safety and Health through Integrated, Facilitated Teams (SHIFT): Stepped-Wedge Protocol for Prospective, Mixed-Methods Evaluation of the Healthy Workplace Participatory Program.** Punnett, L., Nobrega, S., Zhang, Y., Rice, S., Gore, R., & Kurowski, A. BMC Public Health, 20(1), 1–14. 2020. https://www.ncbi.nlm.nih.gov/pmc/articles/PMC7526105/

- **The Elimination of Manual Patient Handling to Prevent Work-Related Musculoskeletal Disorders.** American Nurses Association

(ANA), 2008. https://www.nursingworld.org/~49214e/globalassets/docs/ana/final_pos_stmnt_elimination_manual_patient_handling_031408.pdf

- **The Essential Role of Leadership in Developing a Safety Culture.** The Joint Commission (TJC). Sentinel Event Alert, Issue 57, March 1, 2017. https://www.jointcommission.org/-/media/tjc/documents/resources/patient-safety-topics/sentinel-event/sea_57_safety_culture_leadership_0317pdf.pdf

- **The Importance of Safe Patient Handling to Create a Culture of Safety: An Evidential Review.** Humrickhouse, R., & Knibbe, H. J. Ergon Open J. 9(1): 27–42. 2016 https://benthamopen.com/FULLTEXT/TOERGJ-9-27#

- **The Role of Safe Handling and Mobilization in Reducing Type II Workplace Violence in Healthcare Settings.** Kurowski, A.& El Ghaziri, M. CPH News and Views. Issue #62. UMass Lowell, 2019. https://www.uml.edu/Research/CPH-NEW/News/emerging-topics/News-views-62.aspx

- **Through the Eyes of the Workforce: Creating Joy, Meaning, and Safer Health Care.** The Lucian Leape Institute at the National Patient Safety Foundation. Feb 2013. http://www.ihi.org/resources/Pages/Publications/Through-the-Eyes-of-the-Workforce-Creating-Joy-Meaning-and-Safer-Health-Care.aspx

- **Worker Safety in Hospitals Caring for our Caregivers.** *Website with Multiple Resources.* Occupational Safety and Health Administration (OSHA). https://www.osha.gov/dsg/hospitals/patient_handling.html

- **Worker Safety in Hospitals Safety and Health Management Systems. Tools and Resources.** *Website with Multiple Resources.* Occupational Safety and Health Administration. https://www.osha.gov/dsg/hospitals/mgmt_tools_resources.html

STANDARD 2. IMPLEMENT AND SUSTAIN A SAFE PATIENT HANDLING AND MOBILITY PROGRAM

- **An Inspection Tool and Process to Identify Modifiable Aspects of Acute Care Hospital Patient Care Units to Prevent Work-Related Musculoskeletal Disorders.** Grant, M. P., Okechukwu, C. A., Hopcia, K., Sorensen, G., & Dennerlein, J. T. Workplace Health & Safety, 66(3):144–158. 2018. https://doi.org/10.1177/2165079917718852

- **A Survey of Healthcare Workers on Safe Patient Handling and Mobility Resource Availability, Utilization, and Adherence.** Waltrip, K. Dissertations. 910. 2019. https://irl.umsl.edu/dissertation/910

- **Bariatric Safe Patient Handling and Mobility Guidebook: A Resource Guide for Care of Persons of Size.** Center for Engineering & Occupational Safety and Health (CEOSH), US Department of Veterans Affairs (VA). 2016. http://www.tampavaref.org/safe-patient-handling/implementation-tools.htm

- **Beyond Getting Started: A Resource Guide for Implementing a Safe Patient Handling Program in the Acute Care Setting.** Association of Occupational Health Professional in Healthcare (AOHP), 2014. https://www.aohp.org/aohp/Portals/0/Documents/ToolsForYourWork/free_publications/Beyond%20Getting%20Started%20Safe%20Patient%20Handling%20-%20May%202014.pdf.pdf

- **Current Topics in Safe Patient Handling and Mobility.** American Nurse Today, Sept. 2014. https://www.myamericannurse.com/wp-content/uploads/2014/07/ant9-Patient-Handling-Supplement-821a_LOW.pdf

- **The Facts About Ergonomics: Dispelling Myths: Position Statement.** American Industrial Hygiene Association (AIHA), 2019. https://aiha-assets.sfo2.digitaloceanspaces.com/AIHA/resources/Facts-About-Ergonomics-Dispelling-Myths-Position-Statement_200601_130224.pdf.

- **Guidelines for Nursing Homes: Ergonomics for the Prevention of Musculoskeletal Disorders.** Occupational Safety and Health Administration (OSHA), 2009. https://www.osha.gov/sites/default/files/publications/final_nh_guidelines.pdf

- **Guideline for Safe Patient Handling: Evidence Table.** Association of periOperative Registered Nurses (AORN), 2017. https://www.aorn.org/-/media/aorn/guidelines/evidence-rating-and-tables/sphm_evidence_table.pdf?la=en&hash=65CD0922A47F76C1A7AD9AFED04C9616

- **Guideline for Safe Patient Handling and Movement.** In Guidelines for Perioperative Practice. Denver, CO: AORN, Inc; 2021. *(For purchase)* https://aornguidelines.org/guidelines/content?sectionid=192587418&view=book

- **Healthcare Workers—Home Health.** *Website with Multiple Resources.* National Institute for Occupational Safety and Health (NIOSH). https://www.cdc.gov/niosh/topics/healthcare/homehealthcare.html

- **Home Healthcare.** *Website with Multiple Resources.* The Occupational Safety and Health Administration (OSHA). https://www.osha.gov/home-healthcare

- **Implementation Works Findings for a Six Year Program of Research Safe Patient Handling and Mobility.** Powell-Cope, G. Presentation at the Healthcare Ergonomics Conference, Portland OR. September 2014. https://www.tampavaref.org/SPH-Files/Healthcare_Ergonomics_Conference_September_2014_FINAL.pdf

- **Implementation of Safe Patient Handling in the US Veterans Health System: A Qualitative Study of Internal Facilitators' Perceptions.** Elnitsky, C. A., Powell-Cope, G., Besterman-Dahan, K. L., Rugs, D., & Ullrich, P. M. *Worldviews on Evidence-Based Nursing,* 12(4), 208–216.2015. https://www.nursingcenter.com/ce_articleprint?an=00000446-201811000-00023

- **Improving Patient and Worker Safety: Opportunities for Synergy, Collaboration and Innovation.** The Joint Commission

(TJC), 2012. http://www.jointcommission.org/assets/1/18/TJC-ImprovingPatientAndWorkerSafety-Monograph.pdf

- **ISO/TR 12296:2012: Ergonomics—Manual Handling of People in the Healthcare Sector.** International Organization for Standardization (ISO). (For purchase) https://www.iso.org/standard/51310.html

- **Long Term Care Interest Group.** *Website with Multiple Resources.* Association for Safe Patient Handling Professionals (ASPHP). https://asphp.org/long-term-care-interest-group/

- **Optimizing a Business Case for Safe Health Care: An Integrated Approach to Safety and Finance.** Website with multiple resources. Institute for Healthcare Improvement (IHI). http://www.ihi.org/resources/Pages/Tools/Business-Case-for-Safe-Health-Care.aspx

- **OSHA and Worker Safety Handling with Care Practicing: Safe Patient Handling.** The Joint Commission (TJC), 2017. https://www.jcrinc.com/-/media/jcr/jcr-documents/about-jcr/osha-alliance/pages_from_ecn_20_2017_08-2.pdf?db=web&hash=E471E08D9AC494C0D2C740FD4103DACD

- **Patient-Handling Injuries: Risk Factors and Risk-Reduction Strategies.** Fragala et al. American Nurse Today, 11(5):40–43. 2016. https://www.myamericannurse.com/wp-content/uploads/2016/05/Patient-Handling-Safety-426b.pdf

- **Patient Handling and Mobility Assessments.** Matz, M. et al. Facility Guidelines Institute, 2nd ed., 2019. https://www.fgiguidelines.org/wp-content/uploads/2019/10/FGI-Patient-Handling-and-Mobility-Assessments_191008.pdf

- **Physical Therapist and Physical Therapist Assistants in Safe Patient Handling And Mobility.** HOD P06-19-24-10. APTA's position statement on safe patient handling and mobility, 2019. https://www.apta.org/apta-and-you/leadership-and-governance/policies/pt-and-pta-safe-patient-handling

- **Safe Patient Handling Algorithms.** National Association of Orthopedic Nurses (NAON), 2016. *(For purchase)* http://www.orthonurse.org/p/bl/et/blogaid=926.

- **Safe Patient Handling and Mobility Guidebook.** Center for Engineering & Occupational Safety and Health (CEOSH), VA, 2016. http://www.tampavaref.org/safe-patient-handling/implementation-tools.htm

- **Safe Patient Handling and Mobility (SPHM).** *Website with Multiple Resources.* National Institute for Occupational Safety and Health (NIOSH). https://www.cdc.gov/niosh/topics/safepatient/default.html

- **Safe Patient Handling and Movement.** Website with multiple resources. The American Physical Therapy Association (APTA). https://www.apta.org/patient-care/interventions/safe-patient-handling

- **Safe Patient Handling: Preventing Musculoskeletal Disorders in Nursing Homes.** Occupational Safety and Health Administration (OSHA), 2012. https://www.osha.gov/Publications/OSHA3708.pdf

- **Safe Patient Handling Programs: Effectiveness and Cost Savings.** Occupational Safety and Health Administration (OSHA), 2016. https://www.osha.gov/Publications/OSHA3279.pdf

- **Safe Patient Handling Position Statement.** Association of Occupational Health Professionals in Healthcare (AOHP), 2012. Revised 2014, Reviewed 2020. https://aohp.org/aohp/Portals/0/Documents/NewsAndEvents/Press%20Release/AOHP%20positon%20statements%202-%202020.pdf

- **Safe Patient Handling and Mobility Tip Sheet.** AIHA/OSHA Alliance. American Industrial Hygiene Association (AIHA), 2014. https://aiha-assets.sf02.digitaloceanspaces.com/AIHA/resources/OSHA-Quick-Tips-on-SPHM_Final-Mar2014.pdf

- **Safety Risk Assessment Toolkit | A Process to Mitigate Risk [CHD Tools].** The Center for Health Design. (2014, 2017). https://www.healthdesign.org/sra

- **Saving our Backs: Safe Patient Handling and Mobility for Home Care** Beauvais, A., & Frost, L. Home Healthcare Now, 32(7), 430–434. 2014. https://nursing.ceconnection.com/ovidfiles/00004045-201407000-00008.pdf

- **SPHM in the Pandemic Resources**. *Website with Multiple Resources.* Association for Safe Patient Handling Professionals (ASPHP). https://asphp.org/resources-tools/sphm-in-the-pandemic-resources/

- **SPHM Solutions Everywhere for Everyone: In the Best Interest of the Patient and Their Caregivers. (2021).** Hilton, T. Veterans Health Administration. https://www.publichealth.va.gov/docs/employeehealth/SPHM-Solutions-Everywhere-for-Everyone.pdf#

- **Summaries of Our Applied Research: Patient Handling.** Website with multiple resources. The OHIO State University Spine Research Institute. https://spine.osu.edu/ergonomics/applied-research-patient-handling

- **The Rapid Entire Body Assessment (REBA).** Hignett, S., & McAtamney, L. Applied Ergonomics, 31(2), 201–205. 2000. An Ergonomics risk assessment tool to evaluate type of unpredictable working postures found in health care and other service industries e.g., during patient handling. The tool can be used before and after an intervention to demonstrate that the intervention has worked to lower the risk of musculoskeletal injury. *Access via Cornell University Ergonomics. Website.* http://ergo.human.cornell.edu/ahREBA.html

- **The Use of Lift Teams in Safe Patient Handling Programs—A Summary.** Washington State Hospital Association, 2014. http://www.wsha.org/wp-content/uploads/Compentency_Guide_for_SPH_Champions.pdf

- **Worker Safety in Hospitals Caring for our Caregivers**. *Website with Multiple Resources.* Occupational Safety and Health Administration (OSHA). https://www.osha.gov/dsg/hospitals/patient_handling.html

- **Safe Lifting and Movement of Nursing Home Residents.** DHHS (NIOSH) Publication Number 2006-117. (February 2006).https://www.cdc.gov/niosh/docs/2006-117/default.html

STANDARD 3. INCORPORATE ERGONOMIC DESIGN PRINCIPLES TO PROVIDE A SAFE ENVIRONMENT OF CARE

- **An Inspection Tool and Process to Identify Modifiable Aspects of Acute Care Hospital Patient Care Units to Prevent Work-Related Musculoskeletal Disorders.** Grant, M. P., Okechukwu, C. A., Hopcia, K., Sorensen, G., & Dennerlein, J. T. Workplace Health & Safety, 66(3):144–158. 2018. https://doi.org/10.1177/2165079917718852
- **Bariatric Safe Patient Handling and Mobility Guidebook: A Resource Guide for Care of Persons of Size.** Center for Engineering & Occupational Safety and Health (CEOSH), US Department of Veterans Affairs (VA). 2016. http://www.tampavaref.org/safe-patient-handling/implementation-tools.htm
- **Patient Handling and Mobility Assessments.** Matz, M. et al. Facility Guidelines Institute (FGI). 2nd ed. 2019. https://www.fgiguidelines.org/wp-content/uploads/2019/10/FGI-Patient-Handling-and-Mobility-Assessments_191008.pdf
- **PtD-NIOSH Prevention Through Design.** National Institute for Occupational Safety and Health (NIOSH). 2013. https://www.cdc.gov/niosh/topics/ptd/
- **Safe Patient Handling and Mobility Guidebook.** Center for Engineering & Occupational Safety and Health (CEOSH), VA. 2016. http://www.tampavaref.org/safe-patient-handling/implementation-tools.htm
- **Safety Risk Assessment Toolkit | A Process to Mitigate Risk [CHD Tools].** The Center for Health Design. (2014, 2017). https://www.health-design.org/sra

STANDARD 4. SELECT, INSTALL, AND MAINTAIN SAFE PATIENT HANDLING AND MOBILITY TECHNOLOGY

- **Americans With Disabilities (ADA) Access to Medical Care for Individuals With Mobility Disabilities—Use of SPH Equipment in Clinics.** Department of Health and Human Services Office for Civil Rights (HHS OCR), 2010. https://www.hhs.gov/sites/default/files/ocr/civilrights/understanding/disability/adamobilityimpairmentsgudiance.pdf
- **Bariatric Safe Patient Handling and Mobility Guidebook: A Resource Guide for Care of Persons of Size.** Center for Engineering & Occupational Safety and Health (CEOSH), US Department of Veterans

Affairs (VA). 2016. http://www.tampavaref.org/safe-patient-handling/implementation-tools.htm

- **Can Exoskeletons Reduce Musculoskeletal Disorders in Healthcare Workers?** Posted on November 4, 2020 by Liying Zheng, PhD. NIOSH Science blog. National Institute for Occupational Safety and Health (NIOSH). https://blogs.cdc.gov/niosh-science-blog/2020/11/04/exoskeletons-hc/

- **Corrective and Preventive Maintenance Checklist for Ceiling Mounted Patient Lifts.** VA. 2016. https://www.publichealth.va.gov/employeehealth/patient-handling/index.asp

- **Do Lift Slings Significantly Change the Efficacy of Therapeutic Support Surfaces?** Brienza D, Deppisch M, Gillespie C, et al. Washington, DC: National Pressure Injury Advisory Panel (NPIAP), 2015. https://cdn.ymaws.com/npiap.com/resource/resmgr/white_papers/1a._npuap-lift-sling-white-p.pdf

- **Exoskeletons and Occupational Health Equity.** Posted on December 14, 2020 by Lakshmi D. Robertson et al. NIOSH Science blog. National Institute for Occupational Safety and Health (NIOSH).https://blogs.cdc.gov/niosh-science-blog/2020/12/14/exoskeletons-health-equity/

- **Facility and Patient Needs Assessment: Worker Safety in Hospitals.** Occupational Health and Safety Administration (OSHA) (n.d.). https://www.osha.gov/dsg/hospitals/needs_assessment.html

- **Guideline for Safe Patient Handling and Movement.** In Guidelines for Perioperative Practice. Denver, CO: AORN, Inc; 2021. *(For purchase)* https://aornguidelines.org/guidelines/content?sectionid=192587418&view=book

- **Healthcare Recipient Sling and Hanger Bar Compatibility Guidelines**. American Association for Safe Patient Handling and Movement (ASPHM), 2016. https://aasphm.org/wp-content/uploads/AASPHM-Sling-Hanger-Bar-Guidelines-2016.pdf

- **How Much SPH Equipment Do You Need? Workplace Safety Initiative.** Oregon Association of Hospitals and Health Systems (OAHHS), 2014. https://oahhs.org/assets/Safe%20Patient%20Handling/How%20Much%20SPM%20Equipment%20Do%20you%20NeedEnos.pdf

- **Human Factors Program and Medical Device Use Resources.** Information for Health Care Professional, Manufacturers and Consumers. *Website with Multiple Resources.* US Food & Drug Administration (FDA). http://www.fda.gov/MedicalDevices/DeviceRegulationandGuidance/HumanFactors/default.htm

- **Installation and Relocation Checklist for Ceiling Mounted Patient Lifts**. VA. 2016. https://www.publichealth.va.gov/employeehealth/patient-handling/index.asp

- **ISO10535:2006 Hoists for the Transfer of Disabled Persons—Requirements and Test Methods.** International Organization for

Standardization (ISO). *(For purchase)* https://www.iso.org/standard/32155.html

- **ISO/TR 12296:2012: Ergonomics—Manual Handling of People in the Healthcare Sector.** International Organization for Standardization (ISO). *(For purchase)* https://www.iso.org/standard/51310.html
- **Manufacturer and User Facility Device Experience (MAUDE) Database.** Reports of adverse events involving medical devices. Searchable data base provided. US Food & Drug Administration (FDA). http://www.accessdata.fda.gov/scripts/cdrh/cfdocs/cfmaude/textsearch.cfm
- **Medical Devices—General Hospital Devices and Supplies: Patient Lifts.** *Website with Multiple Resources.* US Food & Drug Administration (FDA). http://www.fda.gov/MedicalDevices/ProductsandMedicalProcedures/GeneralHospitalDevicesandSupplies/ucm308622.htm
- **MedSun: Medical Product Safety Network.** Adverse event reporting program designed to promote reporting of medical device issues by healthcare organizations. Searchable data base provided. US Food & Drug Administration (FDA). http://www.fda.gov/medicaldevices/safety/medsunmedicalproductsafetynetwork/default.htm
- **Patient Handling and Mobility Assessments.** Matz, M. et al. Facility Guidelines Institute (FGI). 2nd ed. 2019. https://www.fgiguidelines.org/wp-content/uploads/2019/10/FGI-Patient-Handling-and-Mobility-Assessments_191008.pdf
- **Patient Handling (Lifting) Equipment Coverage & Space Recommendations.** VA. 2016. https://www.publichealth.va.gov/employee-health/patient-handling/index.asp
- **Patient Lifts.** US Food & Drug Administration (FDA), 2014. https://www.fda.gov/media/88149/download
- **Safe Patient Handling and Mobility Guidebook.** Center for Engineering & Occupational Safety and Health (CEOSH), VA. 2016. http://www.tampavaref.org/safe-patient-handling/implementation-tools.htm
- **Safe Patient Handling Equipment Purchasing Checklist.** Enos, L. *International Journal of Safe Patient Handling and Movement,* 10 (1): 13–36. 2018. Can be accessed from the Oregon Association of Hospitals and Health Systems (OAHHS) Workplace Safety Initiative webpage. https://oahhs.org/assets/Safe%20Patient%20Handling/SPH%20Equipment%20%26%20Sling%20Purchasing%20Checklist%202018.pdf or from the Oregon Coalition for Healthcare Ergonomics (OCHE) website.https://www.hcergo.org/wp-content/uploads/2018/09/Equipment-checklist- for-Enos-workshop-int-SPHM-conf-2018.pdf
- **Safety Risk Assessment Toolkit | A Process to Mitigate Risk [CHD Tools].** The Center for Health Design. (2014, 2017). https://www.health-design.org/sra
- **SPHM Solutions Everywhere for Everyone: In the Best Interest of the Patient and Their Caregivers. (2021).** Hilton, T. Veterans Health

Administration. https://www.publichealth.va.gov/docs/employeehealth/
SPHM-Solutions-Everywhere-for-Everyone.pdf#

- **Technological Change in Health Care Delivery: Its Drivers and Consequences for Work & Workers.** Litwin, A.S. Berkeley: UC Berkeley Labor Center, 2020.https://laborcenter.berkeley.edu/wp-content/uploads/2020/07/Technological-Change-in-Health-Care-Delivery.pdf

STANDARD 5. ESTABLISH A SYSTEM FOR EDUCATION, TRAINING, AND MAINTAINING COMPETENCE

- **Applied Ergonomics for Nurses and Health Care Workers.** Training video. Oregon OSHA, 2004. https://www.youtube.com/watch?v=Vy8T8 BUAbE4&feature=youtu.be
- **Applied Ergonomics for Nurses and Health Care Workers—A Guide for Instructors.** Oregon OSHA, 2004. https://osha.oregon.gov/edu/grants/train/Documents/instructor-guide-safe-patient-handling-in-health-care.pdf
- **Bariatric Safe Patient Handling and Mobility Guidebook: A Resource Guide for Care of Persons of Size.** Center for Engineering & Occupational Safety and Health (CEOSH), US Department of Veterans Affairs (VA). 2016. http://www.tampavaref.org/safe-patient-handling/implementation-tools.htm
- **Current Topics in Safe Patient Handling and Mobility**. American Nurse Today, Sept. 2014. https://www.myamericannurse.com/wp-content/uploads/2014/07/ant9-Patient-Handling-Supplement-821a_LOW.pdf
- **Ergonomics in Healthcare: A Continuing Education Program for Nurses, Nursing Assistants and Healthcare Managers**, U Mas—Lowell, 2018. www.uml.edu/Research/CPH-NEW/nurse-education/ergonomics/
- **Injured Nurses.** The National Public Radio Special Series, 2015. http://www.npr.org/series/385540559/injured-nurses
- **Quick Tips for Safe Patient Handling and Mobility**. American Industrial Hygiene Association (AIHA) and The Occupational Safety and Health Administration (OSHA), 2014.
  - *English:* https://aiha-assets.sfo2.digitaloceanspaces.com/AIHA/resources/OSHA-Quick-Tips-on-SPHM_Final-Mar2014.pdf
  - *Spanish:* https://aiha-assets.sfo2.digitaloceanspaces.com/AIHA/resources/Quick-Tips-on-SPHM-Spanish-OSHA-review-6-27-14_FINAL.pdf
- **Patient Handling and Mobility Assessments.** Matz, M. et al. Facility Guidelines Institute (FGI). 2nd ed. 2019. https://www.fgiguidelines.org/wp-content/uploads/2019/10/FGI-Patient-Handling-and-Mobility-Assessments_191008.pdf

- **Safe Patient Handling Nursing School Curriculum Module.** National Institute for Occupational Safety and Health (NIOSH), 2009. http://www.cdc.gov/niosh/docs/2009-127/
- **Safe Patient Handling (SPH) Training Competency Guide for SPH Champions.** Washington State Hospital Association, 2014. http://www.wsha.org/wp-content/uploads/Compentency_Guide_for_SPH_Champions.pdf
- **Time for Safe Patient Handling and Mobility.** Training video. Washington State Hospital Association, 2015. https://vimeo.com/132744617
- **Training Curriculum for Homecare Workers. Caring for Yourself While Caring for Others.** DHHS (NIOSH) Publication Number 2015-102. National Institute for Occupational Safety and Health (NIOSH), 2015. https://www.cdc.gov/niosh/docs/2015-102/default.html
- **Safe Patient Handling and Movement: Guidance for Health Care Workers.** Online training course. The American Physical Therapy Association (APTA), 2011. https://learningcenter.apta.org/student/MyCourse.aspx?id=ba540aab-937f-485e-a6ce-48b7fbcb3d3f&programid=dcca7f06-4cd9-4530-b9d3-4ef7d2717b5d
- **Safe Patient Handling and Mobility Guidebook.** Center for Engineering & Occupational Safety and Health (CEOSH), VA., 2016. http://www.tampavaref.org/safe-patient-handling/implementation-tools.htm
- **Sample-Safe Patient Handling Observation Survey-Audit.** Workplace Safety Initiative. Oregon Association of Hospitals and Health Systems (OAHHS), 2014. https://oahhs.org/assets/Safe%20Patient%20Handling/Worker-Safety_Sample-SPH-audit-with-patient-feedback.pdf
- **The Caretaker Crisis. Investigating Work Related Injuries in Healthcare.** Video. WA State Department of Labor & Industries, 2015. https://lni.wa.gov/safety-health/safety-research/completed-projects/safe-patient-handling

STANDARD 6. INTEGRATE PATIENT-CENTERED SAFE PATIENT HANDLING AND MOBILITY ASSESSMENT, PLAN OF CARE, AND USE OF SAFE PATIENT HANDLING AND MOBILITY TECHNOLOGY

- **Bariatric Safe Patient Handling and Mobility Guidebook: A Resource Guide for Care of Persons of Size.** Center for Engineering & Occupational Safety and Health (CEOSH), US Department of Veterans Affairs (VA). 2016. http://www.tampavaref.org/safe-patient-handling/implementation-tools.htm
- **Guideline for Safe Patient Handling and Movement.** In Guidelines for Perioperative Practice. Denver, CO: AORN, Inc; 2021. *(For purchase)* https://aornguidelines.org/guidelines/content?sectionid=192587418&view=book

- **ISO 10535:2006 Hoists for the Transfer of Disabled Persons—Requirements and Test Methods**. International Organization for Standardization (ISO). *(For purchase)* https://www.iso.org/standard/32155.html
- **ISO/TR 12296:2012: Ergonomics—Manual Handling of People in the Healthcare Sector.** International Organization for Standardization (ISO). (For purchase) https://www.iso.org/standard/51310.html
- **Patient Handling and Mobility Assessments.** Matz, M. et al. Facility Guidelines Institute (FGI). 2nd ed. 2019. https://www.fgiguidelines.org/wp-content/uploads/2019/10/FGI-Patient-Handling-and-Mobility-Assessments_191008.pdf
- **Safe Patient Handling Algorithms**. National Association of Orthopedic Nurses (NAON), 2016. *(For purchase)* http://www.orthonurse.org/p/bl/et/blogaid=926.
- **Safe Patient Handling and Mobility Guidebook.** Center for Engineering & Occupational Safety and Health (CEOSH), VA. 2016. http://www.tampavaref.org/safe-patient-handling/implementation-tools.htm
- **Scoring System Helps Choose Approaches and Devices for Safely Moving Patients, Leading to Fewer Staff Injuries and Lost Work Days.** Agency for Healthcare Research and Quality (AHRQ), 2012. https://innovations.ahrq.gov/profiles/scoring-system-helps-choose-approaches-and-devices-safely-moving-patients-leading-fewer
- **The Bedside Mobility Assessment Tool 2.0**. Boynton, T., Kumpar, D., & VanGilder, C. American Nurse Journal 15(7):18–22. https://www.myamericannurse.com/wp-content/uploads/2020/06/an7-Mobility-618.pdf
- **The VA Safe Patient Handling and Mobility Mobile App for HealthCare Professionals, Veterans and families. US Department of Veterans Affairs** (VA). https://mobile.va.gov/app/safe-patient-handling

STANDARD 7. INCLUDE SAFE PATIENT HANDLING AND MOBILITY IN REASONABLE ACCOMMODATION AND POST-OCCUPATIONAL INJURY RETURN TO WORK

- **Americans with Disabilities Act of 1990. Public Law No. 101-336.** *United States statutes at large* 104 (1990): 327. https://www.govinfo.gov/content/pkg/STATUTE-104/pdf/STATUTE-104-Pg327.pdf
- **Effectiveness of Workplace Interventions in Return-to-Work for Musculoskeletal, Pain-Related and Mental Health Conditions: An Update of the Evidence and Messages for Practitioners.** Cullen, K. L. et al. Journal of Occupational Rehabilitation 28(1):1–15. 2018. https://www.ncbi.nlm.nih.gov/pmc/articles/PMC5820404/

- **Elements of Ergonomics Programs. Step 6: Promote Worker Recovery through Health Care Management and Return-to-Work.** *Website with Multiple Resources* National Institute for Occupational Safety and Health (NIOSH). https://www.cdc.gov/niosh/topics/ergonomics/ergoprimer/step6.html
- **Guidance on Returning to Work.** US Department of Labor Occupational Safety and Health Administration (OSHA). OSHA 4045-06, 2020. https://www.osha.gov/Publications/OSHA4045.pdf
- **Information and Technical Assistance on the Americans with Disabilities Act.** *Website with Multiple Resources.* Department of Health and Human Services Office for Civil Rights (HHS OCR). https://www.ada.gov/
- **OSHA Injury and Illness Recordkeeping and Reporting Requirements.** Occupational Safety and Health Administration (OSHA). https://www.osha.gov/recordkeeping.
- **Worker Compensation Return to Work Guidebook.** Society Insurance, 2014. http://www.societyinsurance.com/assets/1/AssetManager/Return%20to%20Work.pdf

STANDARD 8. ESTABLISH A COMPREHENSIVE EVALUATION SYSTEM

- **A Survey of Healthcare Workers on Safe Patient Handling and Mobility Resource Availability, Utilization, and Adherence.** Waltrip, K. Dissertation. 910. 2019. https://irl.umsl.edu/dissertation/910
- **Bariatric Safe Patient Handling and Mobility Guidebook: A Resource Guide for Care of Persons of Size.** Center for Engineering & Occupational Safety and Health (CEOSH), US Department of Veterans Affairs (VA). 2016. http://www.tampavaref.org/safe-patient-handling/implementation-tools.htm
- **Beyond Getting Started: A Resource Guide for Implementing a Safe Patient Handling Program in the Acute Care Setting.** Association of Occupational Health Professional in Healthcare (AOHP), 2014. https://www.aohp.org/aohp/Portals/0/Documents/ToolsForYourWork/free_publications/Beyond%20Getting%20Started%20Safe%20Patient%20Handling%20-%20May%202014.pdf.pdf
- **Evaluation of a Continued Safe Patient and Handling Program.** Daily, M. K. Dissertation. *UMASS-Amherst, 2014.* https://scholarworks.umass.edu/cgi/viewcontent.cgi?article=1035&context=nursing_dnp_capstone
- **Guidelines for Nursing Homes: Ergonomics for the Prevention of Musculoskeletal Disorders.** Occupational Safety and Health Administration (OSHA), 2009. https://www.osha.gov/ergonomics/guidelines/nursinghome/final_nh_guidelines.html

- **Guideline for Safe Patient Handling and Movement.** In Guidelines for Perioperative Practice. Denver, CO: AORN, Inc; 2021. *(For purchase)* https://aornguidelines.org/guidelines/content?sectionid=192587418&view=book
- **Implementation Works Findings for a Six Year Program of Research Safe Patient Handling and Mobility.** Powell-Cope, G. Presentation at the Healthcare Ergonomics Conference, Portland OR. September 2014. https://www.tampavaref.org/SPH-Files/Healthcare_Ergonomics_Conference_September_2014_FINAL.pdf
- **Implementation of Safe Patient Handling in the US Veterans Health System: A Qualitative Study of Internal Facilitators' Perceptions.** Elnitsky, C. A., Powell-Cope, G., Besterman-Dahan, K. L., Rugs, D., & Ullrich, P. M. *Worldviews on Evidence-Based Nursing*, *12*(4), 208–216. 2015. https://www.nursingcenter.com/ce_articleprint?an=00000446-201811000-00023
- **Improving Patient and Worker Safety: Opportunities for Synergy, Collaboration and Innovation.** The Joint Commission (TJC), 2012. http://www.jointcommission.org/assets/1/18/TJC-ImprovingPatientAndWorkerSafety-Monograph.pdf
- **Interaction of Health Care Worker Health and Safety and Patient Health and Safety in the US Health Care System: Recommendations From the 2016 Summit.** Loeppke, R. et al. American College of Occupational and Environmental Medicine (ACOEM) Position Statement. Journal of Occupational and Environmental Medicine, 59(8), 803–813. 2017. http://www.acoem.org/uploadedFiles/Public_Affairs/Policies_And_Position_Statements/Guidelines/Position_Statements/Interaction_of_Health_Care_Worker_Health_and.17.pdf
- **Leading a Culture of Safety: A Blueprint for Success.** American College of Healthcare Executives (ACHE). Institute for Healthcare Improvement NPSF, 2017. https://www.osha.gov/shpguidelines/docs/Leading_a_Culture_of_Safety-A_Blueprint_for_Success.pdf
- **Linking Worker Health and Safety with Patient Outcomes.** Gibson, K., Costa, B., & Sampson, A. WorkSafe Victoria (WSV). The Institute of Safety, Compensation and Recovery Research (ISCRR). 2017. http://www.iscrr.com.au/__data/assets/pdf_file/0006/1321719/Evidence-Review_Linking-worker-health-and-safety-with-patient-outcomes.pdf
- **Long Term Care Interest Group.** *Website with Multiple Resources.* Association for Safe Patient Handling Professionals (ASPHP). https://asphp.org/long-term-care-interest-group/
- **Measuring Best Practices for Workplace Safety, Health, and Well-Being. The Workplace Integrated Safety and Health Assessment.** Sorensen, G., Sparer, E., Williams, J. A., Gundersen, D., Boden, L. I., Dennerlein, J. T., . . . & Pronk, N. P. Journal of Occupational and Environmental Medicine, 60(5), 430–439. 2018. https://dl.uswr.ac.ir/bitstream/

- **Missed Nursing Care.** Agency for Healthcare Research and Quality (AHRQ). AHRQ PSNet Patient Safety Primer. Updated Sept. 2019. https://psnet.ahrq.gov/primer/missed-nursing-care
- **Nurses Create a Culture of Patient Safety: It Takes More Than Projects.** Morath, J. American Nurses Association (ANA), *OJIN*. September 3, 2015. http://ojin.nursingworld.org/MainMenuCategories/ANAMarketplace/ANAPeriodicals/OJIN/TableofContents/Vol-16-2011/No3-Sept-2011/Nurses-Create-a-Culture-of-Patient-Safety.aspx#:~:text=Nurses%20play%20an%20essential%20role%20in%20developing%20the,provide%20leadership%20to%20strengthen%20the%20culture%20of%20safety
- **Occupational Injury and Illness Data—Federal and State.** US Bureau of Labor Statistics. http://www.bls.gov/iif/
- **Optimizing a Business Case for Safe Health Care: An Integrated Approach to Safety and Finance.** *Website with Multiple Resources.* Institute for Healthcare Improvement (IHI). http://www.ihi.org/resources/Pages/Tools/Business-Case-for-Safe-Health-Care.aspx
- **Patient Handling and Mobility Assessments.** Matz, M., et al. Facility Guidelines Institute (FGI). 2nd ed. 2019. https://www.fgiguidelines.org/wp-content/uploads/2019/10/FGI-Patient-Handling-and-Mobility-Assessments_191008.pdf
- **Recommended Practices for Safety and Health Programs.** OSHA 3885. Occupational Safety and Health Administration (OSHA), 2016. https://www.osha.gov/Publications/OSHA3885.pdf
- **Safety and Health Through Integrated, Facilitated Teams (SHIFT): Stepped-Wedge Protocol for Prospective, Mixed-Methods Evaluation of the Healthy Workplace Participatory Program.** Punnett, L., Nobrega, S., Zhang, Y., Rice, S., Gore, R., & Kurowski, A. BMC Public Health, 20(1), 1–14. 2020. https://www.ncbi.nlm.nih.gov/pmc/articles/PMC7526105/
- **Safe Lifting and Movement of Nursing Home Residents.** DHHS (NIOSH) Publication Number 2006-117 (February 2006). https://www.cdc.gov/niosh/docs/2006-117/default.html
- **Safe Patient Handling and Mobility Guidebook.** Center for Engineering & Occupational Safety and Health (CEOSH), VA, 2016. http://www.tampavaref.org/safe-patient-handling/implementation-tools.htm
- **Safe Patient Handling and Mobility (SPHM).** *Website with Multiple Resources.* National Institute for Occupational Safety and Health (NIOSH). https://www.cdc.gov/niosh/topics/safepatient/default.html
- **Safe Patient Handling and Movement.** *Website with Multiple Resources.* The American Physical Therapy Association (APTA). https://www.apta.org/patient-care/interventions/safe-patient-handling
- **Safe Patient Handling—A Self-Assessment Checklist.** The Occupational Safety and Health Administration (OSHA). 2013. https://www.osha.gov/dsg/hospitals/documents/3.8_SPH_self-assessment_508.pdf

- **Safe Patient Handling Program—Gap Analysis Checklist 2018**. Oregon Association of Hospitals and Health Systems (OAHHS) Workplace Safety Initiative. 2018. https://oahhs.org/assets/Safe%20Patient%20Handling/ SPH%20Program%20Gap%20Analysis%20tool%20with%20survey%20 2018.pdf
- **The Importance of Safe Patient Handling to Create a Culture of Safety: An Evidential Review.** Humrickhouse, R., & Knibbe, H. J. *The Ergonomics Open Journal* 9(1): 27–42. 2016. https://benthamopen.com/ FULLTEXT/TOERGJ-9-27#
- **The Role of Safe Handling and Mobilization in Reducing Type II Workplace Violence in Healthcare Settings**. Kurowski, A. & El Ghaziri, M. CPH News and Views Issue #62. UMass Lowell, 2019. https://www. uml.edu/Research/CPH-NEW/News/emerging-topics/News-views-62. aspx
- **Worker Safety in Hospitals Caring for Our Caregivers.** *Website with Multiple Resources.* Occupational Safety and Health Administration (OSHA). https://www.osha.gov/dsg/hospitals/patient_handling.html
- **Worker Safety in Hospitals Safety and Health Management Systems. Tools and Resources.** *Website with Multiple Resources.* Occupational Safety and Health Administration. https://www.osha.gov/dsg/hospitals/ mgmt_tools_resources.html

Glossary

ancillary/support staff for SPHM—Individuals whose work provide necessary support to the SPHM program. This may include consultants and staff members from departments such as risk management, safety, infection prevention, occupational health, transportation, security, activity direction, recreational therapy, creative art therapy, environmental services, laundry, volunteers, engineering, biomedical engineering, facilities, morgue, funeral home, purchasing, and contracting.

assessment for SPHM—Use of a scoring or other system to examine and evaluate the physical, mental, cognitive, medical, and/or environmental conditions of a healthcare consumer to determine appropriate SPHM methods, technology, and supplies. Assessment for SPHM may be an interprofessional activity, with collaboration from several disciplines.

assisted products—Hoists for the transfer of disabled persons—Requirements and test methods. ISO 10535:2021—International Organization for Standardization. This document specifies safety-related design requirements and test methods for the manufacture of mechanical lifts and accessories, such as slings, used in moving and handling healthcare consumers. The standard is recognized as a voluntary consensus standard for medical products by the US Food and Drug Administration; thus, to be able to distribute or sell their SPHM products in the United States, manufacturers must meet the requirements of this ISO standard.

bariatric healthcare consumer—See *individual of size.*

care plan—See *plan of care.*

community settings—Non-hospital settings where healthcare consumers are provided medical care and consultations, and/or interventions are performed. These settings include, but are not limited to, the healthcare consumer's home, long-term care, rehabilitation centers, assisted living facilities, group homes, healthcare clinics, outpatient facilities, schools, prisons, congregant facilities, and day care.

competence—An expected, measurable, and confirmed level of performance that integrates knowledge, skills, abilities, and judgment, based on established scientific knowledge and expectation for practice.

continuum of care—Description of the entire range of healthcare that can be provided, from the beginning of care to the end of care, encompassing all care modalities, and through all phases of care and environments of care.

culture of safety—Core values and behaviors resulting from a collective and sustained commitment by organizational leadership, managers, and healthcare workers to emphasize safety over competing goals.

delegation—The transfer of responsibility for the performance of a task from one individual to another, while retaining accountability for the outcome. The decision of whether or not to delegate is based upon professional judgment concerning the condition of the healthcare consumer, the competence of the individual being delegated to, and the degree of supervision that will be required.

education—The transfer of information to others in order to raise awareness and increase understanding of the subject. Includes relaying of information during orientation and in-service education.

employer—The healthcare organization, agency, system, corporation, business, or person(s) that employ or contract with the healthcare worker, at all levels of the continuum of care. The term *organization* is used interchangeably in these standards.

environment of care—Any environment in which health care is being provided, such as pre-hospital care, hospital units, surgery, dental, rehabilitation, long-term care, assisted living, home care, hospice, ambulatory care, occupational health, group homes, schools, correctional facilities, morgues, and other similar settings.

ergonomic design principles—A systematized approach to prevent or reduce hazards that might result in musculoskeletal injuries and other related illnesses, fatalities, and exposures by including ergonomic and human factors considerations in all construction and remodeling designs.

ergonomics—The scientific discipline concerned with the understanding of interactions among humans and other elements of a work system. In healthcare, such a system would include care tasks performed for the healthcare consumer, other work tasks not involving healthcare consumers, the physical and organizational environment where work is performed, and the tools used to help perform the work. Ergonomics encompasses the knowledge of human physical and cognitive abilities and limitations as applied to the design of work systems, organizations, job tasks, equipment, building components, and environments to prevent or reduce the risk of error and musculoskeletal and other injuries/disorders.

essential physical functions—The physical duties that a healthcare worker must be able to perform for a specific job, with or without reasonable accommodation.

evaluation—A comprehensive system to assess or analyze SPHM program status, using staff performance, healthcare consumer outcome metrics, and a mechanism to provide organizational leadership and key stakeholders with results from these analyses.

formative evaluation—A method of assessing the worth of a program while the program activities are in progress. A formative evaluation focuses on process.

healthcare consumer—In the context of these standards, they are individuals who are receiving health care that involves assistance with handling and mobility. This definition is inclusive of patients, clients, residents, students, individuals living in community settings, and others as appropriate.

healthcare worker—In the context of these standards, any person involved in the provision of care to a healthcare consumer that involves the tasks of moving, handling, and mobilization, at any level in the continuum of care. Examples of healthcare workers include, but are not limited to, nurses, nursing assistants, resident assistants, home health aides, direct care workers working in community settings, occupational therapists, physical therapists, therapist assistants, radiology and surgical technologists, medical assistants, morgue personnel, emergency medical technicians, paramedics, hospital transporters, physicians, dentists, schoolteachers, and para-educators. Patient families and volunteer caregivers are also included.

high-risk tasks—For the purposes of these standards, patient handling and mobility tasks characterized by biomechanical and postural stressors imposed on the healthcare worker. These tasks are considered high risk based on the frequency of repetitive motions, duration of stress, and the degree of musculoskeletal stress imposed by the task. A high-risk task is a care activity that can result in musculoskeletal injuries in healthcare workers.

home care—Services provided to individuals and families in their homes or residences. The care may be either supportive or custodial in nature, such as assistance with bathing, dressing, or feeding; or skilled care that requires the interventions of a licensed healthcare professional such as a nurse, therapist, or physician. Home care is unique among healthcare settings in that the healthcare worker is a guest in the healthcare consumer's home; therefore, the healthcare consumer and family have much greater control over how the plan of treatment is delivered.

individual of size (IOS)—For SPHM purposes, individuals of size (IOS) are defined as those who have a BMI that exceeds 30 or who have a body weight of 300 pounds or greater. IOS also includes people who are tall and/or muscular and not necessarily obese; thus, body habitus (height, body shape, and weight and height distribution) is considered when determining if a healthcare consumer is an "individual of size." These criteria represent thresholds for instituting expanded capacity SPHM technology and techniques. IOS replaces the previously used terms "bariatric patient" and "patient of size".

injury—For the purposes of these standards, damage or harm to the healthcare worker or healthcare consumer as a result of patient care, handling, movement, and/or mobilization.

interprofessional—Reliant on the overlapping knowledge, skills, and abilities of each professional team member. Interprofessionalism can drive synergistic effects by which outcomes are enhanced and become more comprehensive than a simple aggregation of the individual efforts of the team members.

long-term care—Medical and nonmedical services provided to people with a chronic illness or disability who cannot care for themselves for long periods of time. Long-term care can be provided at home, in the community, in assisted living facilities, or in nursing homes.

manager/management—Defined for the purpose of these standards as middle and frontline management, such as nurse managers, radiology supervisors, charge nurses, and operational leaders (among others), who ensure application of policies and procedures.

manual handling—Lifting, lowering, pushing, pulling, repositioning, transferring, or in some way moving or supporting a healthcare consumer or body part of a healthcare consumer without mechanical assistance.

mobility—Defined for the purpose of these standards as the maintenance or increase in physical activity of a healthcare consumer.

mobilize—To facilitate physical movement or a change in position of a healthcare consumer, either of the body or of a body part, from one place or position to another. Mobilization can engage the healthcare consumer's own capabilities or be passively induced by a healthcare worker and/or technology. For example, a healthcare consumer who is dependent or requires extensive assistance can be mobilized in bed (turned, moved to head of bed) or transferred out of bed to another surface such as a chair. A healthcare consumer with partial weight-bearing capability can be assisted to stand and ambulate. Mobilizing healthcare consumers has been found to decrease negative health outcomes such as pressure injuries, overall weakness, deep vein thrombosis, pneumonia, and urinary tract infections. Using SPHM technology in early and progressive mobility programs promotes preservation of patient functional status and improves clinical outcomes. In the long-term care and home settings, SPHM technology can preserve independence and mobility to improve quality of life.

musculoskeletal disorder (MSD)—Musculoskeletal disorders (MSD) are injuries or disorders of the muscles, nerves, tendons, ligaments, joints, cartilage, and spinal discs that can occur in the upper and lower limbs, neck, and back. Examples of MSDs include strains and sprains, tendonitis, bursitis, and spinal disc herniation. MSDs are caused by sudden exertion or prolonged exposure to one or more physical risk factors such as overexertion, awkward postures, repetitive motion, and vibration.

non-punitive environment—An environment that fosters trust to encourage healthcare workers to disclose errors so that the precursors to errors can be better understood and remedied. Healthcare workers know that they are accountable for their actions but will not be held accountable for problems within the system or environment that are beyond their control.

organization—The healthcare organization, agency, system, corporation, business, or person(s) that employ or contract with the healthcare worker at all levels of the continuum of care. The term *employer* is used interchangeably in these standards.

organizational leadership—Defined for the purpose of these standards as the high-level, senior leaders of the employer, such as those in the "C-Suite," the senior leadership team, the chief officer(s), president, vice president(s), or others with significant strategic or operational roles.

patient. See *healthcare consumer*.

patient handling and mobility assessment (PHAMA)—A multidisciplinary, documented systematic process conducted to direct and assist a design team as they incorporate and accommodate appropriate handling and mobility technology in the health care environment, including such for individuals of size and to facilitate healthcare consumer mobilization.

patient handling injury—A healthcare worker injury due to performing handling and mobility activities with healthcare consumers.

peer leader—A staff member who receives special education and training on SPHM and use of SPHM technology. Peer leaders are the SPHM subject-matter expert in their clinical units/areas and share knowledge and skills with coworkers, management, and healthcare consumers. Peer leaders foster knowledge transfer and forge a direct connection between staff and SPHM program goals. This term is commonly used in Veterans Health Administration care settings.

plan of care (SPHM)—An individualized, written, patient-centered handling and mobilization plan developed for each healthcare consumer. It is based on the use of an SPHM assessment or scoring system that generates SPHM technology and techniques that serve the capabilities, needs, and goals of the healthcare consumer. The SPHM plan of care is incorporated into the overall plan of care.

return to work program—A program designed and administered to safely return individuals who have sustained injuries or illnesses to the work environment, in a full or transitional capacity, as quickly as is medically advisable. The goal of the program is to enhance worker recovery and/or rehabilitation, minimize direct and indirect costs associated with work injury or illness, and prevent service interruption.

right of refusal—The right of the healthcare worker to refuse an assignment, or the right of a healthcare consumer to refuse a treatment or the use of SPHM technology.

simulation—A method used to educate and train healthcare professionals to master cognitive, technical, and behavioral skill sets through technologically crafted experiences. Simulation allows the acquisition of clinical skills through deliberate practice rather than an apprentice style of learning. Simulation tools serve as an alternative to real healthcare consumers. A trainee can make mistakes and learn from them without the fear of harming the healthcare consumer.

SPHM—Safe Patient Handling and Mobility. There are various definitions of SPHM in use, but in general, SPHM refers to the application of ergonomics to reduce the risk of injury to healthcare workers and consumers during handling and mobility tasks and enhance the health outcomes of healthcare consumers.

SPHM program—A multifaceted program that uses ergonomic principles to improve the health and safety of healthcare workers and healthcare consumers, and the financial wellbeing of healthcare organizations. SPHM programs include program elements that support the use of SPHM technology, that, in turn, reduce the risk of musculoskeletal disorders (MSDS) and other healthcare worker injuries that are associated with manual lifting, repositioning, and transfers of healthcare consumers. These support structures may include facility program managers, clinical unit/area peer leaders/champions, healthcare recipient assessments, knowledge/information transfer mechanisms (i.e., Safety Huddles), education/training, and others. Such programs enhance health outcomes for healthcare consumers through safe and early mobilization. For healthcare organizations, they reduce costs associated with healthcare worker MSDs, staff turnover, and healthcare consumer outcomes.

subject-matter expert (SME)—A person who exhibits the highest level of expertise in performing a specialized job, task, or skill set. Examples include those with advanced knowledge of SPHM, ergonomics, industrial hygiene, human factors, and biomechanics.

summative evaluation—A method of assessing the worth of a program at the end of the program activities. A summative evaluation focuses on outcomes.

technology—The assistive tools used to facilitate the healthcare worker's performance of high-risk healthcare recipient handling, movement, and mobilization tasks, thus, minimizing the risk of injury to the healthcare consumer and the healthcare worker. Technology may include equipment, devices, accessories, software, and multimedia resources.

technology needs assessment—An assessment done using ergonomic principles of evaluation. The assessment includes evaluation of the physical, mental, and cognitive characteristics of the healthcare consumer or population, and the physical environment of care in which care is being delivered, so as to recommend appropriate SPHM methods and technology.

training—The process of bringing a person to an agreed statement of competency that includes the knowledge, skills, and abilities (KSAs) necessary to achieve successful performance. For SPHM, hands-on practice or simulation applications are critical training modalities.

universal SPHM—The attainment of an organizationally effective and interdisciplinary SPHM program for safely handling and mobilizing healthcare consumers, resulting in safe environments of care for healthcare workers and consumers, exceptional quality of care for healthcare consumers, and facilitation of attainment of the designation of a High Reliability Organization.

Index

A

Accessibility, SPHM technology for, 48

Accidents, in SPHM, 39, 40

Accommodation, in SPHM, 58, 77–78

Accountability, in SPHM, 39, 42, 58, 62

Activities, SPHM, 56

Acute care settings
early mobility programs in, 19
healthcare consumers with ARDS, 3
Hospital Patient Care Units, 68, 72
Safe Patient Handling Program in, 69, 78
SPHM technology in, 2–3

Acute respiratory distress (ARDS), 3

Agency for Health Care Research and Quality (AHRQ), 20, 67, 77, 80

Alzheimer's disease, 15

Ambulatory settings, SPHM programs and technologies, 15

American Association for Safe Patient Handling and Movement (ASPHM), 73

American College of Healthcare Executives (ACHE), 66, 79

American College of Occupational and Environmental Medicine (ACOEM), 66, 79

American Industrial Hygiene Association (AIHA), 69, 71, 75

American Nurses Association (ANA), 37
ANA Quality Conference, 12
culture of safety, 65, 66, 67, 80
"Handle with Care" campaign, 11, 65
SPHM Interprofessional National Standards, see SPHM Interprofessional National Standards
universal SPHM, *see* Universal SPHM

American Physical Therapy Association (APTA), 70, 76, 80

Americans with Disabilities Act (ADA), 62, 77, 78

ANA, *see* American Nurses Association (ANA)

Analysis, in SPHM
cost/benefit, 43

data, evidence-based methods for, 61

Ancillary/support staff for SPHM, 9
competence, 52
culture of safety, 39
defined, 83
education and training, 52
ergonomic design principles, for safe environment of care, 46
implementation and sustainment SPHM programs, 42
responsibilities, 37

Aon, 32, 33

Artificial intelligence (AI), AI-enabled robotic-assistive devices, 26–27

Assessment for SPHM
comprehensive, 42
defined, 83
initial and ongoing, 55
patient-centered
employer standards, 55–56
resources, 76–77
PHAMA, 12, 30, 87
Safety Risk Assessment (SRA), 30
technology needs assessment, 42, 48, 49, 88
Workplace Integrated Safety and Health Assessment, 67, 79

Assisted products-Hoists for the transfer of disabled persons, ISO 10535:2021, 12, 13, 27, 35, 73, 77, 83

Association for Safe Patient Handling Professionals (ASPHP), 12, 13, 70, 71, 79

Association of Occupational Health Professionals in Healthcare (AOHP), 69, 71, 78

Association of periOperative Registered Nurses (AORN), 69

Attitudes, in SPHM, 17

Authority, in SPHM, 42

Automated lift systems, in SMPH, 26

B

Back injuries, incidents of, 11

Bariatric healthcare consumer, *see* Individual of size

Behaviors, in SPHM, 17, 27, 39

Beliefs, in SPHM, 17

Beverly Enterprises, 11

Bureau of Labor Statistics (BLS) data, 1–2

Business case, building and sustaining, 32–33

C

Care and caring
acute care settings, *see* Acute care settings
continuum of care, *see* Continuum of care
environment of care, *see* Environment of care
"Handle with Care" campaign, 11, 65, 70
healthcare consumers, *see* Healthcare consumers
healthcare workers, *see* Healthcare workers
home-based care, *see* Home-based care
long-term care, *see* Long-term care
plan, *see* Plan of care

Caregivers, in SPHM, 68, 71, 74–75, 81

Center for Engineering & Occupational Safety and Health (CEOSH)
Bariatric SPHM Guidebook, 68, 72–73, 75, 76, 78
SPHM Guidebook, 70, 72, 74, 76, 77, 80

Center for Health Design (CHD), 71, 72, 74

Certified Safe Patient Handling Professionals™, 12

Codes of ethics, in SPHM, 62

Collaboration, in SPHM
opportunities for, 66, 69–70, 79
safety culture, 17, 40
SPHM Interprofessional National Standard, 40, 42

Commitment, in SPHM, 17, 39

Communication, in SPHM
with healthcare consumer and family, 56
safety culture, 17, 40
SPHM Interprofessional National Standard, 40, 56, 62

Community settings, in SPHM
considerations for
assessment and plan of care, 56
comprehensive evaluation system, 62
culture of safety, 40

ergonomic design principles, 46
implementation and sustainment SPHM programs, 43
reasonable accommodation, 58
selection, installation, and maintenance, SPHM technology, 49
system for education, training, and maintaining competence, 53
defined, 83

Compensation, in SPHM
claim, cost of, 2, 32, 33
laws, 62

Competencies, in SPHM
defined, 83
safety culture, 17
SPHM Interprofessional National Standards, 52–53
considerations for community settings, 53
employer standards, 52
healthcare worker standards, 52–53

Compliance, in SPHM, 35, 42, 61

Comprehensive evaluation system
resources, 78–81
SPHM Interprofessional National Standards
considerations for community settings, 62
employer standards, 61–62
healthcare worker standards, 62

Construction, SPHM in, 30

Continuous improvement, in SPHM, 17

Continuum of care, in SPHM
defined, 83
healthcare workers from across, 52
program across, 42
safety culture, 17

Conyers, John, Jr., 35

Costs, in SPHM
cost/benefit analysis, 43
healthcare worker injuries, 2, 4, 32, 55, 58
overexertion-related injuries, 2
savings, 71
workers' compensation, 2, 32, 33

COVID-19 pandemic and SPHM, 3–4
telemedicine to deliver care, 27

Culture of safety, in SPHM
creating and maintaining, 40
defined, 84
effective, facilitation, 17

resources, 65–68
SPHM Interprofessional National
  Standards, 39–40
  considerations for community
    settings, 40
  employer standards, 39–40
  healthcare worker standards, 40

D

Data, in SPHM
  analysis, evidence-based methods for, 61
  BLS, 1–2
  collection
    accurate information during, 62
    comprehensive ability, 26
    evidence-based methods for, 61
  employee benchmarking, 32
  sources and measures, 61

Deficiencies, remediation of, 62

Delegation, in SPHM
  defined, 84
  SPHM tasks, 56

Delirium, immobility and, 19

Demographics and characteristics of US
  population, 15

Department of Health and Human
  Services (DHHS), 11, 72, 76, 78, 80

Design, SPHM in, 30

Development, in SPHM
  AI-enabled robotic-assistive devices, 26
  business plan, 30
  comprehensive evaluation system, 61, 62
  culture of safety, 65, 68
  design requirements, 30
  healthcare facilities' documents, 46
  multifaceted ergonomics program, 65
  plan for performance/quality
    improvement, 62
  SPHM programs, 17, 30, 42
  SPHM technology
    for accessibility, 48
    cleaning, disinfection, and
      maintenance, 49
    plan for selection of, 48
    procurement plan, 48
  of standards, 9, 65
  system, for safety of healthcare worker,
    55
  written SPHM program, 42

DHHS Office for Civil Rights (HHS OCR),
  72, 78

Diabetes, 15

Disabled persons, transfer of, 12, 13, 27, 35,
  73–74, 77

Disseminate findings, 81

Division of Occupational Safety and Health
  (DOSH), 11

Documentation, in SPHM
  assisted products—Hoists for the
    transfer of disabled persons, ISO
    10535:2021, 12, 13, 27, 35, 73, 77,
    83
  healthcare facilities, 46
  healthcare worker competence, 52
  of physical limitations or restrictions, 58
  physical mobility during hospitalization,
    19
  resources, 65
  SPHM assessment and plan of care, 55

Durable Medical Equipment (DME), 43

E

Education, in SPHM
  defined, 84
  SPHM Interprofessional National
    Standards, 52–53
    considerations for community
      settings, 53
    employer standards, 52
    healthcare worker standards, 52–53

Electronic beds, 25

Emergency response, SPHM programs and
  technologies, 15

Employees, in SPHM
  benchmarking data, 32
  in learning sessions, 52

Employers, in SPHM
  defined, 84
  of hazards, 40
  SPHM Interprofessional National
    Standards
    assessment and plan of care, 55–56
    comprehensive evaluation system,
      61–62
    culture of safety, 39–40
    ergonomic design principles, 46
    implementation and sustainment
      SPHM programs, 42–43
    reasonable accommodation, 58
    selection, installation, and
      maintenance, SPHM technology,
      48–49

system for education, training, and maintaining competence, 52

Environment of care, in SPHM
  defined, 84
  resources, 72
  SPHM Interprofessional National Standards
    considerations for community settings, 46
    employer standards, 46
    healthcare worker standards, 46

Ergonomic design principles, for safe environment of care
  defined, 84
  resources, 72
  SPHM Interprofessional National Standards
    considerations for community settings, 46
    employer standards, 46
    healthcare worker standards, 46

Ergonomic Guidelines for Manual Material Handling, 11

Ergonomics—Manual Handling of People in the Healthcare Sector, 12, 35, 70, 74, 77

Errors, in SPHM, 5
  culture of safety, 17, 39
  healthcare worker, 27
  medication, 30

Essential physical functions, in SPHM
  defined, 84
  identification, 43

Ethical responsibility, in SPHM, 17

Evaluation, in SPHM
  comprehensive evaluation system
    employer standards, 61–62
    resources, 78–81
  defined, 84

Evidence-based design (EBD) approach, SPHM and, 30

Evidence-based methods for data collection, 61

Exoskeletons, in SPHM, 26, 73

Expected outcomes, in SPHM, 55

F

Facility Guidelines Institute (FGI), 12, 30, 46, 72, 74, 75, 77, 80

Falls, SPHM programs and, 19, 20

Families, in SPHM, 3, 27, 49, 52, 53, 56

Federal Nursing and Healthcare Worker Protection Act, 12

Fixed SPHM technology, 48

Food and Drug Administration (FDA), 12, 73, 74

Formative evaluation, 61, 85

Fragala, Guy, 13

Funding
  to implement and sustain program, 43
  strategies for SPHM technology, 42

G

Gait-related disorders, 26

General Duty clause violations, 35

Goals, in SPHM
  of ANA, 3
  comprehensive evaluation system, 61
  culture of safety, 39
  of design requirements, 30
  implementation and sustainment SPHM programs, 42
  programs, 4–5, 42
  SPHM assessment and plan of care, 55
  technology, 26, 27

Groups, in SPHM
  Advisory Group and Workgroup, 37
  comprehensive evaluation system, 62
  culture of safety, 17
  implementation and sustainment SPHM programs, 42
  long term care interest, 70, 79
  selection, installation, and maintenance, SPHM technology, 48
  of stakeholders, 3, 42, 48, 62

Guidelines for Design and Construction of Health Care Facilities, 30

Guidelines for Nursing Homes— Ergonomics for the Prevention of Musculoskeletal Disorders (OSHA), 11

H

"Handle with Care" campaign, 11, 65, 70

Hazard Alert letters, 35

Hazards, in SPHM
  culture of safety, 17, 39, 40
  employer of, 40
  by OSHA, 35

M

Maintenance, in SPHM
competence, 52–53
considerations for community
settings, 53
employer standards, 52
healthcare worker standards, 52–53
culture of safety, 40
technology
considerations for community
settings, 49
employer standards, 48–49
healthcare worker standards, 49
resources, 72–75

Manager/management
defined, 86
healthcare, 75
SPHM, 4, 17, 39

Manual handling, in SPHM, 12, 30, 35, 70, 74, 77
defined, 86
healthcare worker injuries and, 4
workplace violence, 21

Manufacturer and User Facility Device Experience (MAUDE) database, 74

MedSun, 74

Meetings, in SPHM, 61

Missed nursing care
causative factors for, 21
defined, 20
resources, 67, 80

Mobility
defined, 86
SPHM, *see* Safe patient handling and mobility (SPHM) standards

Mobilization, in SPHM, 19, 68, 81
defined, 86
early and progressive, 19
of healthcare consumers, 12, 20, 30

Monitoring, in SPHM
compliance, 42
healthcare worker injuries, 55, 58
responsibility for, 49

Morbidity rates, US population, 15

MSDs, *see* musculoskeletal disorders (MSDs)

Multidisciplinary team, SPHM and, 30

Musculoskeletal disorders (MSDs)
defined, 86
exoskeletons, 73
focus on, 12
in healthcare worker, 19, 32, 42
incidence rates, 1–2
injuries, 35, 71
prevention, 67–68, 69, 70, 72, 78
rates of, 21
return-to-work for, 77
SPHM program, 19, 88
work- related, 67–68, 72

N

National Association of Orthopedic Nurses (NAON), 70, 77

National Emphasis Program, 35

National Institute for Occupational Safety and Health (NIOSH)
DHHS, 72, 76, 80
Fundamentals of Total Worker Health® Approaches, 65
Healthcare Workers—Home Health, 69
lifting injuries in nurses, 11
PtD-NIOSH Prevention Through Design, 72
SPHM, resources, 65, 69, 70, 72, 73, 76, 78, 80

National Patient Safety Foundation, 68

National Pressure Injury Advisory Panel (NPIAP), 73

Near misses, in SPHM, 17, 40

Needs, SPHM, 1–5
of adult learner, 52
of community settings, 53
facility and patient needs, 73
initial and ongoing assessments, 55–56
for SPHM technology, 27
technology needs assessment, 42, 48, 49, 88
for universal SPHM, 4

Nelson, Audrey, Dr., 11, 65

NIOSH, *see* National Institute for Occupational Safety and Health (NIOSH)

Non-punitive environment
defined, 86–87
SPHM Interprofessional National Standard, 39

Nurse and Health Care Worker Protection Act, 35

Nurses
ANA, *see* American Nurses Association (ANA)
lifting injuries in, 11
RNs, *see* registered nurses (RNs)

Nursing home settings, 70
guidelines for, 11, 69, 78
residents, 21, 72, 80
SPHM technology in, 3

O

Obesity rates, US population, 15

Objectives, in SPHM, 37, 42, 61

Occupational Safety and Health Administration (OSHA)
CAL/OSHA, 11
Guidelines for Nursing Homes, 11
for inpatient healthcare settings, 35
Inspection Guidance for Inpatient Healthcare Settings, 12
National Emphasis Program (NEP), 12
SPHM, resources, 67, 68, 69, 70, 71, 73, 75, 78, 80, 81
vs. Beverly Enterprises, 11

Oregon Association of Hospitals and Health Systems (OAHHS), 73, 74, 76, 81

Organizational leadership, in SPHM, 9, 39, 42, 61, 87

Organizational policy, in SPHM, 39, 56, 62

Organizations, in SPHM
comprehensive evaluation system, 61–62
culture of safety, 39
defined, 87
healthcare, *see* healthcare organizations
priorities, 39
safety culture, 17

OSHA, *see* Occupational Safety and Health Administration (OSHA)

Outcomes, in SPHM, 55, 61–62

Overhead lifts, 25, 26

P

Participation, in SPHM
culture of safety, creating and maintaining, 40
employees, in learning sessions, 52

in organizational decision-making, 4
return-to-work plan, 58
in SPHM program, 43
SPHM technology, selection, 49
technology needs assessment, 49

Patient, *see* healthcare consumer

Patient-centered SPHM assessment
SPHM Interprofessional National Standards
considerations for community settings, 56
employer standards, 55–56
healthcare worker standards, 56

Patient handling and mobility assessment (PHAMA), 12, 30, 87

Patient Handling and Movement Assessments, 12, 30, 46, 80

Patient handling injury, 67, 70, 87

Patient safety, in SPHM, 17

Patient Safety Center of Inquiry (PSCI), 11

Peer leaders, defined, 87

Perceptions, in SPHM, 17

Performance, in SPHM
ergonomics evaluations of, 43
improvement, 61–62
SPHM program, 32
staff, 61–62

Planning, in SPHM, 3, 30
comprehensive evaluation system, 61, 62
for ongoing evaluation, 42
for performance/quality improvement, 62
safe environment of care during new construction and/or renovation, 46
for selection of SPHM technology, 48
SPHM technology procurement plan, 48

Plan of care, SPHM
defined, 87
resources, 76–77
SPHM Interprofessional National Standards
considerations for community settings, 56
employer standards, 55–56
healthcare worker standards, 56

Pneumonia
cause of death, 15
immobility and, 19

Point-of-care training, 52